Innovations
IN PLASTIC SURGERY

Cohesive Gel Implants

Editor: **Ian T. Jackson,** MD, DSc(Hon), FRCS, FRCS(Ed), FACS, FRACS(Hon)
Director, Institute for Craniofacial and Reconstructive Surgery; Chief, Division of
Plastic Surgery, Providence Hospital, Southfield, Michigan

Coeditor: **Claudio De Lorenzi,** BA, MD, FRCS   Medical Director, De Lorenzi Clinic and Silhouette
Cosmetic Laser Clinic; Plastic Surgeon, Department of Surgery, Grand River Hospital,
Kitchener, Ontario, Canada

Contributors: **William P. Adams, Jr., MD**   Associate Clinical Professor, Department of Plastic Surgery,
University of Texas Southwestern Medical Center, Dallas, Texas

Phillip Blondeel MD, PhD   Professor, Department of Plastic and Reconstructive Surgery,
University Hospital, Gent, Belgium

Stefano Bonomi, MD   Resident, Department of Plastic and Reconstructive Surgery,
Istituto Nazionale per lo Studio e la Cura dei Tumori, Milan, Italy

Umberto Cortinovis, MD   Plastic Surgeon, Department of Plastic and Reconstructive
Surgery, Istituto Nazionale per lo Studio e la Cura dei Tumori, Milan, Italy

Bruce L. Cunningham, MD, MS   Program Director, Division of Plastic and Reconstructive
Surgery, University of Minnesota, Minneapolis, Minnesota

Continued.

DISCLOSURE

It is the policy of Ciné-Med to ensure balance, independence, objectivity, and scientific rigor in all its educational programs. Faculty, course directors, and planners participating in an accredited program are required to disclose to the program audience any real or apparent conflict(s) of interest. This pertains to relevant financial relationships within the past 12 months with a commercial interest and the opportunity to affect program content relevant to products or services of that commercial interest. The intent of this policy is to allow for a determination to be made as to whether that relationship may constitute a conflict of interest that must be resolved. Information that a faculty member, course director, or planner (including spouse/partner) has no relevant financial relationships will be provided to the learners. In addition, all faculty members are expected to disclose discussion of any off-label or investigational uses of products.

Dr. William P. Adams, Jr. is the Medical Director for Mentor Corporation cohesive gel implant trial, is an Investigator for Inamed and Mentor Corporation cohesive gel implant IDE trials, and is on the speaker's bureau for commercial sponsors for Inamed Academy. **Dr. Bruce L. Cunningham** receives grant/research support from Mentor Corporation and Inamed, and is a consultant for Mentor Corporation. **Dr. Claudio De Lorenzi** receives grant/research support from and is on the speaker's bureau for Medicis, Mentor Corporation, and QMed. Dr. De Lorenzi also discusses the off-label or investigational use of silicone breast implants (not FDA approved). **Dr. Dennis C. Hammond** receives financial/material support from Surgical Specialty and discusses off-label or investigational use of products related to the sale of the Dermaspan tissue expander.

Drs. Phillip Blondeel, Stefano Bonomi, Umberto Cortinovis, José Luis Martín del Yerro, Paulo Miranda Godoy, João Carlos Sampaio Góes, Renata Sampaio Góes, Ian T. Jackson, Alan Landecker, Maurizio Nava, Rolf R. Olbrisch, Angela Pennati, and **Andrea Spano** have no relevant financial relationships to disclose.

Dr. José Luis Martín del Yerro now has a consulting agreement with Mentor Medical Systems, CV which was not the case at the time of printing.

José Luis Martín del Yerro, MD   Director del Instituto de Cirugía Plástica Martín del Yerro; Jefe de Servicio de Cirugía Plástica del Hospital Quirón Madrid, Madrid, Spain

Paulo Miranda Godoy, MD   Resident, Department of Surgery, Faculdade de Medicina da Universidade de Santo Amaro, São Paulo, SP, Brazil

João Carlos Sampaio Góes, MD, PhD   Faculdade de Medicina da Universidade de São Paulo; Diretor Técnico Cientifico, Instituto Brasileiro de Controle do Câncer, São Paulo, SP, Brazil

Renata Sampaio Góes, MD   Resident, Department of Gynecology and Obstetrics, Faculdade de Medicina da Universidade de Santo Amaro, São Paulo, SP, Brazil

Dennis C. Hammond, MD   Center for Breast and Body Contouring, Grand Rapids, Michigan

Alan Landecker, MD   Plastic Surgeon, Clínica Sampaio Góes, São Paulo, SP, Brazil

Maurizio Nava, MD   Department Head, Department of Plastic and Reconstructive Surgery, Istituto Nazionale per lo Studio e la Cura dei Tumori, Milan, Italy

Rolf R. Olbrisch, MD   Formerly Professor, Department Head, Department of Plastic Surgery, Florence Nightingale Hospital, Duesseldorf; Department of Plastic Surgery, MEOCLINIC, Berlin, Germany

Angela Pennati, MD   Plastic Surgeon, Department of Plastic and Reconstructive Surgery, Istituto Nazionale per lo Studio e la Cura dei Tumori, Milan, Italy

Andrea Spano, MD   Plastic Surgeon, Department of Plastic and Reconstructive Surgery, Istituto Nazionale per lo Studio e la Cura dei Tumori, Milan, Italy

Future Topics

- Patient Safety

- Fixation Devices

- Nonsurgical Cosmetic Treatments

Innovations

CONTACT INFORMATION

Issues of *Innovations in Plastic Surgery* are available by contacting:
Quality Medical Publishing, Inc.
2248 Welsch Industrial Court
St. Louis, MO 63146, USA
Telephone: 314-878-7808
Fax: 314-878-9937
Email: customerservice@qmp.com

Information on advertising rates may be obtained by contacting QMP Advertising and Sales at 314-878-7808.

Innovations in Plastic Surgery (ISSN 1547-3376) is a periodical published by QMP. Corporate and editorial offices: 2248 Welsch Industrial Court, St. Louis, MO 63146, USA. Periodicals postage paid at St. Louis, MO 63146, and at additional mailing offices.

Send address changes to:
Innovations in Plastic Surgery
Quality Medical Publishing, Inc.
2248 Welsch Industrial Court
St. Louis, MO 63146, USA

Statements and opinions expressed in articles, editorials, and roundtables published in *Innovations in Plastic Surgery* are not necessarily those of the editors, publisher, board of directors, or trustees. Publishing of advertisements in *Innovations in Plastic Surgery* is not a guarantee, warranty, or endorsement of any products or services therein by Quality Medical Publishing, Inc., authors, or editors.

Innovations
IN PLASTIC SURGERY

Cohesive Gel Implants

Volume 1 • Number 3 • 2007

Contents

Innovations in Plastic Surgery (ISSN 1547-3376)
is a periodical published by Quality Medical Publishing, Inc., 2248 Welsch Industrial Court, St. Louis, MO 63146, USA.

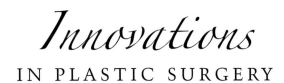

Innovations

IN PLASTIC SURGERY

Cohesive Gel Implants

Volume 1 • Number 3 • 2007

CME Information

Learning Objectives
After reading this publication, participants should be able to:
• Describe how to use cohesive gel implants for different body types
• Explain the step-by-step techniques for various breast reconstruction procedures
• Discuss the current status of cohesive gel implants in the marketplace
• Identify ways to embrace new devices and products while ensuring the safety of patients

Target Audience
This publication is intended for plastic surgeons, residents, and other allied health professionals.

Accreditation
Ciné-Med, Inc. is accredited by the Accreditation Council for Continuing Medical Education (ACCME) to provide continuing medical education for physicians.

Ciné-Med, Inc. designates this educational activity for a maximum of 4 AMA PRA Category 1 Credit(s)™. Physicians should only claim credit commensurate with the extent of their participation in the activity.

The accreditation period for this material is September 2006 to August 2008.

Commercial Support
This activity is supported by an unrestricted educational grant from Mentor.

Obtaining Credit
United States and international readers: To receive CME credit for the completion of this activity, mail or fax the completed Registration (with payment), Post Test, and Evaluation Forms located at the back of this publication to: Ciné-Med, Inc., CME Department, 127 Main Street North, Woodbury, CT 06798, Fax: 203-263-4839. A certificate will be sent via regular mail.

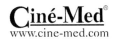

www.cine-med.com

Evolutionary Development of Cohesive Gel Implants: A New Era in Implant Technology

Ian T. Jackson, MD

Cohesive gel implants represent a positive advance in the evolution of breast implant technology. Although cohesive silicone gel is not new technology, having been used in implants since the mid-1980s, the use of the word *cohesive* to describe this gel is relatively recent and refers to the solid consistency of the gel compared with the more liquid fill that was used in some silicone gel implants in the early 1970s. In this context *cohesive* means that the silicone fill is not liquid or semiliquid; it is a solid unit that maintains its softness, holds together uniformly, and retains a natural feel that greatly resembles that of natural breast tissue. The development of cohesive gel implants can best be understood by reviewing the evolution of silicone breast implants.

BACKGROUND

In 1963 the silicone gel implant was introduced by Cronin and Gerow.[1] This first-generation device had a very thick shell with thick seams around the edge; it contained a firm, dense gel. In response to surgeons' requests for thinner, more natural-feeling implants, a second generation of implants was developed and introduced in the 1970s. These second-generation devices had very thin shells with a thin, almost liquid silicone gel filling. The fragile shells proved to be susceptible to rupture with potential for gel leakage. The third generation of implants, introduced in the mid-1980s, sought to address problems associated with the first two generations of implants. These implants were similar to devices manufactured today by the major implant manufacturers. Today's devices have thicker silicone shells with a barrier layer to inhibit gel bleed through the shell; the gel contained within this shell is cohesive and acts as a unit, holding together firmly. Cohesive gel implants have lower rates of rupture and contracture than earlier models, with significantly reduced potential for gel diffusion or bleeding through the shell.

The concept of cohesive gel implants can be traced to the Replicon (Surgitek), an anatomically shaped, polyurethane-coated, silicone-filled implant that was popular in the 1980s. Early results using this implant were very good, but there were long-term problems with polyurethane degradation. Once the polyurethane was gone, the remaining thin, pliable shell could not maintain the implant shape, causing weakening and visible folds that eventually resulted in rupture and silicone leak. In addition to the effects of gravity, constrictive forces acted on the implant to deform its initial anatomic shape.

Tebbetts[2] is credited with introducing the concept that both the shell and its contents contribute to implant shape. This idea has influenced subsequent research, leading to the development of what we now call *cohesive gel implants.* By adding a crosslinker to the silicone in different amounts, manufacturers discovered that they could vary the softness of the material. From this, a soft implant filler was created that maintains its shape after molding. This gel is different from what we have seen with standard implants, where the silicone sinks to the bottom of the implant when it is held up and, when implanted, the implant shape is controlled by the tissue surrounding it. The concept of preventing this from happening was a great step forward in breast implant surgery. Unfortunately, because of the 1992 moratorium on silicone gel implants in the United States, further U.S. development ceased, and progress for bringing this development into clinical use has taken place in Europe and the rest of the world.

During the past decade cohesive silicone gel implants have been used extensively in Europe. As a result of this activity, large series can now be reported that document the efficacy of these devices, which have become the gold standard for breast implants used outside the United States.

CHARACTERISTICS OF THE COHESIVE GEL IMPLANT

The consistency of cohesive gel implants contributes to their appeal and long-term effectiveness. These implants have a firmer texture than the standard gel implants formerly available in the United States. If one is cut in half, or if a preshaped area is removed with scissors, there is no gel extrusion, even if the implant is squeezed. Thus even with rupture the shape is maintained and there is no evidence of gel migration. This phenomenon results from more crosslinking during the manufacture of the gel. Another advantage is that these implants may last longer than other implants.

It must be understood that these are *not* regular gel implants. They offer significant advantages over previous generations. They are long-lasting and maintain their shape after implantation, which may be round or anatomic. The shape is stable over time. No matter what position the patient assumes, the shape remains constant. Conventional implants fail in the fold areas; these implants do not form folds, and even if the shell fails, there is no significant gel migration. In a standard implant, the shape tends to be controlled by the capsule; in cohesive gel implants, the implant controls the shape—thus most are anatomically shaped. The gel consistency ranges from soft (I) to medium (II) to firm (III). It is the firm type that is used most frequently. The breast may be somewhat firmer with a firm implant, but the shape is well maintained, and these implants have found great favor among patients and their partners. Obviously, with softer, less cohesive gels, the implant shape is less stable. An additional modification is that anatomic teardrop implants are textured, which increases friction and prevents the implant from rotating—an essential element in the design of this implant.

Although implant rupture is rare (one Swedish study of several thousand implants reported only a single rupture[1]), it is important to know what happens if one of these devices should rupture. If a rupture occurs, migration of gel is unlikely because of the consistency of the gel, which has been characterized as having a "gummy bear" consistency. Thus if migration occurred, it would be in microscopic amounts. It also seems likely that microscopic migration can occur through the shell, but this does not appear to cause problems.

If rupture occurs it is difficult to diagnose, and evaluation by mammography or MRI may be necessary. From the studies and data available, it appears that the silicone stays inside the capsule. Furthermore, scientific evidence has clearly established that silicone is not related to any health problems. Thus a ruptured implant is not a cause for concern, apart from the aesthetic issues that need to be addressed.

PUBLISHED REPORTS

Numerous reports in the world literature emphasize the potential value of cohesive gel implants. In 2001 Niechajev[3] reported excellent results with these devices. He noted that the margin for error with these implants is small and reported on a new implant design that he had developed using an anterior marking suture and a posterior fixing plate. Fruhstorfer et al[4] placed contour profile gel (CPG) breast implants in 35 patients, 10 of which were cosmetic and 25 of which were reconstructive. Patient satisfaction with breast shape was excellent; 85% of breasts were soft, and there were no significant aesthetic complications. Heden et al,[5] who have the world's most extensive experience with anatomic cohesive gel implants, stated that these implants can produce very predictable results with a high degree of patient satisfaction. Chantal et al[6] presented a case in which a cohesive gel implant was anchored to the chest wall with 3-0 braided polyester sutures. Reoperation at 1 week and MRI after 6 months showed no evidence of silicone leakage. This was a significant contribution. Graf et al[7] in 2003 reported on 263 patients with cohesive gel implants placed in the subfascial plane. They noted that there was no evidence of palpable edges. With subpectoralis implantation, there was no distortion of pectoralis movement even with larger implants of 310 cc. Capsule formation (Baker II) was seen in six patients (2.3%). There was unilateral displacement in eight patients, of which three required surgery. Mira,[8] in a comprehensive 2003 survey comparing cohesive gel implants with standard implants, noted the advantages of the cohesive devices and commented how surprising it was that, despite more than a half century of experience with breast implants, it has taken so long to recognize that they are more than a substitute for volume—they also play a key role in providing breast contour and shape.

These studies reflect worldwide experience with cohesive gel implants. Unfortunately, since the FDA moratorium on silicone gel implants in 1992, the United States has not been able to actively participate in the revolution that is taking place in implant technology. We have been largely limited to saline-filled implants, and as a result have fallen behind our international colleagues. At the moment there are three ongoing studies in the United States: first-time augmentation, revision of breast augmentation, and breast reconstruction following mastectomy. It is hoped that the large prospective studies underway in the United States will lead to FDA approval of these implants in the near future, thereby giving U.S. surgeons the ability to offer patients the cohesive silicone gel implants that represent the state of the art today and are the gold standard of implant technology.

CONCLUSION

Cohesive gel implants offer potential for improving long-term results of breast surgery. Some of the benefits of these implants include the following:

- They are available in three consistencies, graded I, II, and III. As the consistency becomes thicker, the profile increases from low to moderate to increased moderate to high.
- They maintain shape regardless of the patient's position.
- They do not form folds, and thus there is decreased likelihood of failure.
- If a shell fails, there is little likelihood of gel migration.
- An implant controls the shape of the breast and therefore the shape will not change even with significant trauma. This stability increases with the thicker gel types.

REFERENCES

1. Cronin TD, Gerow FJ. Augmentation mammaplasty: A new "natural feel" prosthesis. In Broadbent TR, ed. Transactions of the Third International Congress of Plastic Surgery. Amsterdam: Excerpta Medica, 1964.
2. Tebbetts JB. Dimensional Augmentation Mammaplasty Using the BioDimensional System. Santa Barbara, CA: McGhan Medical, 1994.
3. Niechajev I. Mammary augmentation by cohesive silicone gel implants with anatomic shape: Technical considerations. Aesth Plast Surg 25:397-403, 2001.
4. Fruhstorfer BM, Hodgson EL, Malata CM. Early experience with an anatomical soft cohesive silicone gel prosthesis in cosmetic and reconstructive breast surgery. Ann Plast Surg 53:526-542, 2004.
5. Heden P, Jernbeck J, Hober M. Breast augmentation with anatomical cohesive gel implants: The world's largest current experience. Clin Plast Surg 28:531-552, 2001.
6. Chantal M, Melis P, Marco R. Suturing of a textured breast implant filled with cohesive gel to prevent dislocation. Scand J Plast Reconstr Surg Hand Surg 37:236-238, 2003.
7. Graf RM, Bernardes A, Rippel R, et al. Subfascial breast implant: A new procedure. Plast Reconstr Surg 111:904-908, 2003.
8. Mira J. Anatomic asymmetric prostheses: Shaping the breast. Aesthetic Plast Surg 27:94-99, 2003.

Cohesive Breast Implants: Characteristics and Crosslinking Properties

Bruce L. Cunningham, MD, MS

Gel-filled silicone implants have been in the marketplace for more than 30 years, having been introduced in the 1960s. They have gone through many iterations during this time, from round devices with Teflon patches on them, to form-stable devices undergoing premarket evaluation today. Plastic surgeons are frequently asked by patients and even insurance and regulatory agencies how the devices in clinical practice today are different from those used in the past. Surgeons are also subjected to new-device marketing campaigns containing a combination of scientific and qualitative language that can be confusing. Understanding some of the history of the devices' development, as well as some of the technical differences among them, will help place the shaped devices into perspective.

GENERATIONS OF GEL IMPLANTS

The evolution of silicone-based breast implants was described by Peters et al[1] in their seminal article of 1997, in which they identified three different "generations" of these devices. Other reports have reaffirmed this generational development.[2-4] Still other investigators cite the addition of texturing and anatomic shapes as evidence of additional generational development of these devices instead of refinements to existing devices. Regardless, most would agree that these gel-filled devices have evolved and that the current generation of cohesive gel implants offers distinct advantages over earlier versions.

First-generation implants featured thick shells and a firm gel and were produced until approximately 1979. Second-generation devices were significantly different from their predecessors, with thin shells and a thin, less viscous gel inside. In some instances, loss of shell integrity resulted in the gel freely flowing out of the implant into the capsule, with the shell collapsing into it. This produced a characteristic "linguine" sign in MRI examinations.[5] The shell wall was permeable to the short-chain structure of the gel, and when it diffused through the shell it was called gel bleed, detectable as a filmy layer on the exterior of the implant.

The current generation of breast implants is characterized by firmer gel and thicker, multilayer shells with barrier coats, resulting in extremely low gel bleed. These devices represent a dramatic departure from second-generation implants. The crosslinking of the gel is so complete that if the implant is cut in half, none of the gel flows out.

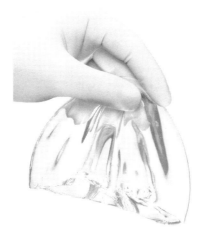

FIG. 1 Mentor Smooth Round Memory Gel implant cut in half.

Because of the characteristic "stickiness" of the gel, these implants are referred to as *cohesive*, meaning that the contents hold together and do not disperse when the shell is broken (Fig. 1). However, despite the increased firmness, these implants do not generally fracture. Although there were overlaps among different manufacturers when they abandoned generation two and moved to generation three, the latter have been in use for almost 20 years. There have been improvements and refinements in manufacturing techniques, but no significant design difference in generation three devices. The current generation of implants features low-bleed gel technology, which may explain why the implants do not seem to have high levels of capsular contracture as seen in early generations.

CHARACTERISTICS AND CROSSLINKING PROPERTIES

Although there are subtly different levels of cohesion among the current-generation implants that are available through FDA-sponsored trials, depending on the desired clinical characteristics and use, the basic characteristics remain the same. Generally, greater crosslinking of the gel results in a firmer, more form-stable device. When this is coupled with an asymmetric shell, unique shapes can be created for different clinical situations. Each manufacturer has taken its own approach to current-generation devices.

For example, Mentor uses an international scale to differentiate cohesive products. *Cohesive I*™ refers to the current round gel products being used in the Adjunct and Round Memory Gel studies currently under review by the FDA. *Cohesive II*™ is a slightly more firm gel used internationally in round gel implants. *Cohesive III*™ is the most firm option, and it is used in the Contour Profile Gel (CPG) product. The Mentor CPG device, the Inamed Style 410 introduced in 1993, and the less crosslinked Style 410 Soft Touch are the most crosslinked and are form-stable asymmetrical devices. These implants have textured shells to help maintain rotational stability.

Because of their ability to create and sustain a shape, these devices are referred to as *anatomic*. Although the data are still being analyzed, there are trade-offs for using the more firm anatomic gel products: They are more palpable, they require more precise surgical technique, and they run the risk of rotation. Different techniques, such as a longer incision, must be used for their implantation. These anatomic gels may represent a good option for patients with specific needs, such as those who need an implant to define breast shape (reconstruction or thin-tissue augmentation patients), but for patients with existing breast tissue, a round silicone implant is also an excellent choice. The surgeon must evaluate the benefits against the risks of the shaped devices and make the best choice for the patient.

However, there do appear to be disadvantages to too much crosslinking. Under extreme localized stress, firmer gels can fail along fracture planes *(gel fracture)*. There have been published reports of gel fractures in the most heavily crosslinked devices.[6] Gel fracture causes the shape of a device to become distorted, sometimes to the point that the implanted breast becomes misshapen. This type of device failure does not involve a ruptured shell, but a reoperation may be necessary to achieve a properly shaped breast mound. Clinicians have reported very few instances of this type of failure (rarely postimplantation, most commonly during insertion), and manufacturers are continuing to closely monitor returned devices for this type of device complaint.[6] A longer incision helps avoid gel fracture and overcome the wall friction associated with these textured devices.

Minor differences in the characteristics of current-generation implants can make significant differences in clinical behavior. For example, there are only two substantive differences between the Mentor Round Memory Gel™ and CPG™ cohesive breast implant devices: The firmness of the silicone gel filler and the contour shape. The difference in shape is controlled by the shape of the shell that surrounds the silicone gel filler, which in turn is determined by the mandrel on which the shell is formed during manufacture. The difference in firmness between the Round Memory Gel and the CPG is the result of a slightly higher crosslink density in the gel filler of the CPG product. This produces a firmer, more shape-retaining gel.

Crosslinking and Implant Firmness

A chemical crosslink is formed when two reactive sites on a crosslinker molecule attach, through chemical reaction, to two separate polymer chains containing sites that can react with the crosslinking molecule. A link is thus formed through chemical reactions between the bridging molecule (crosslinker) and two polymer chains (Fig. 2). The greater the number of crosslinks (crosslink density) the more firm a gel is. In other words, a structural property relationship is established between the chemical and physical characteristics of the material.

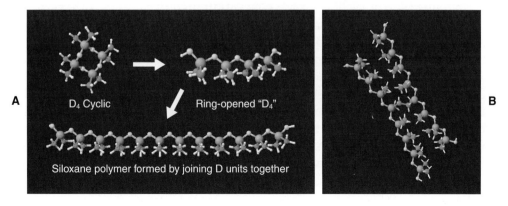

FIG. 2   A, Before crosslinking. **B,** After crosslinking.

The two reactive moieties that combine to form the crosslinks are silicon hydride (SiH) on the shorter crosslink molecules and vinyl groups that are pendant to (attached to) the polymer chains. The silicon hydride groups are internal to the shorter bridging molecules (the crosslinker). The pendant vinyl groups are spaced along the longer polymer chains. The firmness of the silicone gel filler depends directly on the number of crosslinks between the polymer chains, and, therefore, on the amount of crosslinker included in the formulation before the reaction between the silicone hydride (crosslinker molecule) and the polymer chains with the vinyl pendant groups. This means simply that, for a given set of polymers in a gel formulation, the *sole* determinant of gel firmness is the amount of crosslinker included in the formulation.

The implications of these technical details can be illustrated by research from one of the manufacturers. Mentor has demonstrated that crosslink density is the only discernible difference between Round Memory Gel and CPG devices by measuring physical and chemical properties of those devices. The data confirm that the physical properties (ultimate tensile properties, impact resistance, and cyclic fatigue results) of the shells of the two product families are statistically the same (Jerry Barbor, Mentor Corporation, personal communication, 2006). This is expected because the chemical components and processes for making the shells are essentially the same. Stated simply, the chemical bonds and the relative numbers of those bonds per unit volume of shell that are formed during the manufacture of the shells are identical for both families of products. The only differences in the shells of the two families are that the CPG devices have a contoured shape, and the texturing layer is slightly more porous and has a somewhat less amorphous silica reinforcing material than the shells of the Round Memory Gel family.

Similarly, the only difference between the gel filler of the CPG and Round devices is that the CPG gel formulation contains a slightly higher level of crosslinker relative to the vinyl polymer than does the Round. This means that the kinds of chemical bonds in the gel that are formed during the manufacture of the devices are the same for both product families. There is simply slightly more of the crosslink bonds in the gel filler of the CPG devices. Table 1 shows that the crosslink characteristics are similar for both Mentor and Inamed products.

Comparative chemical characterization of the silicone gel from Mentor Round and CPG devices has been undertaken, and Inamed's competitive offerings have also been well characterized. Chemical analysis reveals that the total extractable content of Mentor's gel fillers for both the Round Memory Gel and CPG devices is essentially identical. In addition, the content of individual low-molecular-weight (LMW) cyclic siloxane compounds is also comparable.

The measured LMW cyclic siloxane concentrations in Inamed's corresponding devices *should be* essentially the same, based on data presented to the FDA in April of 2004. The conclusion that can be drawn from the foregoing is that the chemical constituents of the Mentor and Inamed products are similar. One can therefore speculate with a fair degree of certainty that the significant difference between the less cohesive devices and the more cohesive devices in the Inamed product lines is the crosslink density, as is the case with Mentor's devices.

We know that the greater firmness of the Mentor CPG devices compared with the Round devices is created by a simple increase of the crosslinker in the gel formulation, and this difference does not manifest significantly in the chemical characteristics of the filler. However, the difference in cohesiveness can be evaluated from physical measure-

TABLE 1   Crossover Modulus of Mentor and Inamed Silicone Gel Breast Implant Fillers (dynes/cm^2)

Mentor		Inamed	
Memory Gel (Round)	CPG (Contour)	Style 110 (Round)	Style 410 (Contour)
1242	2468	873	2999

ments of the modulus using rheology. The crossover modulus is directly proportional to the cohesiveness or stiffness of the filler. Typical crossover modulus data from samples of devices from each family are presented in Table 1.

The difference in crosslink density between the Mentor product families is considered slight. Based on nominal formulations, the theoretical portion of total vinyl moieties involved in the crosslinking of Round devices is approximately 11.3%, compared with approximately 14.5% for CPG devices. It is interesting to note that the less cohesive Inamed Style 110 has a lower crossover modulus (is less firm) than the corresponding Mentor Round product. The Inamed Style 410 has a higher crossover modulus (is more firm) than the corresponding Mentor CPG product. Nevertheless it should be apparent that the crossover modulus for these products represents a continuum of cohesiveness from the same generation of implants.

CONCLUSION

Most of the world today has embraced cohesive gel devices as the gold standard for breast implant surgery, whereas the U.S. experience has been limited to FDA clinical trials. However, FDA approval of these devices is on the horizon, and U.S. surgeons will soon gain access to them. The issue to address then will be whether the differences in shape and firmness really present a significant advantage to plastic surgeons and their patients. We should be able to answer this question more completely once the preapproval studies are complete, and the data are reported. More importantly, we will ultimately have a great deal of clinical data showing how these implant design changes are incorporated, not into the practices of expert researchers, but into the practices of the average plastic surgeon who chooses to use them.

REFERENCES

1. Peters W, Smith D, Fornasier V, et al. An outcome analysis of 100 women after explantation of silicone gel breast implants. Ann Plast Surg 39:9, 1997.
2. Collis N, Sharpe DT. Silicone gel-filled breast implant integrity: A retrospective review of 478 consecutively explanted implants. Plast Reconstr Surg 105:1979, 2000.
3. Hölmich LR, Friis S, Fryzek JP, et al. Incidence of silicone breast implant rupture. Arch Surg 138:801, 2003.
4. Hölmich LR, Kjøller K, Fryzek JP, et al. Self-reported diseases and symptoms by rupture status among unselected Danish women with cosmetic silicone breast implants. Plast Reconstr Surg 111:723, 2003.
5. Gorczyca DP, Debruhl ND, Mund DF, et al. Linguine sign at MR imaging: Does it represent the collapsed silicone implant shell? Radiology 191:576, 1994.
6. Brown MH, Shenker R, Silver SA. Cohesive silicone gel breast implants in aesthetic and reconstructive breast surgery. Plast Reconstr Surg 116:768, 2005.

Editorial Commentary

Dr. Cunningham has produced a very succinct review of the present situation regarding cohesive gel implants. He points out the advantages of these implants but also adds a word of caution that they must be carefully assessed over time, and an objective evaluation needs to be made to be absolutely certain that these implants are superior to saline-filled implants. It is beneficial to have a certain degree of caution before jumping into deep waters and emerging with some significant problem. This is a very useful article, because it is a prelude to those that describe the experiences of many authors who use this type of implant. In the clinical situation there are certainly pitfalls that largely can be avoided by using proper techniques. It is useful to pay attention to the information in this article.

Ian T. Jackson, MD

Of all the evolutions of breast implants, the second generation is probably the most troublesome one. However, both the first-generation and the troublesome second-generation devices are quickly becoming extinct as patients with these implants show up for replacement surgery.

The latest generation of implants is notable for having a sandwiched barrier layer of polydimethylsiloxane (PDMS), with phenyl groups along the chain, that does a reasonable job of stopping gel bleed. Today's silicone gels contain a nonreactive PDMS fluid that is more than 10,000 mW and trapped in the three-dimensional crosslink network. Gel bleed today is miniscule compared with the old gels and is not composed of short-chain segments. Dr. Cunningham also points out the problem of gel fracture, which is discussed in other articles in this issue.

Many doctors may not be aware of how these implants are produced—manufacturers still rely heavily on handwork to make them. Over the last few years, Mentor has developed the first completely mechanized equipment that can manufacture implant shells with remarkable consistency. By mechanization, these companies can create better, more consistent products of higher quality and more stringent tolerances. This is definitely a win-win arrangement for all concerned.

Materials testing methods are typically used to assess batches of products to ensure that they meet specifications. It is probably not necessary for surgeons to know the technical details of the rheology tests that are done, however Dr. Cunningham points out that the crossover modulus may be used to put a number to the degree of firmness. The absolute value of the number is not important of course, but the rank order of the devices is interesting and correlates well with my clinical experience. Yes, the 410 devices are stiffer than the CPG devices, and the soft touch devices are less stiff than the CPG devices. The information of the degree of stiffness is of value in this regard, and perhaps manufacturers should publish these standardized ASTM numbers on their specification sheets.

Finally, I agree that these devices represent the gold standard of breast augmentation. It remains to be seen whether the devices will be used appropriately when they become generally available in the United States. It is my hope that the U.S. plastic surgery societies and the FDA will agree on an implementation path that includes clinical instruction for surgeons, ensuring that patients get the best devices possible using a best practices model.

Claudio De Lorenzi, BA, MD

Form-Stable Cohesive Gel Implants: Advantages and Technical Essentials

William P. Adams, Jr., MD

The advent of form-stable cohesive gel implants represents a significant *device-related* advance in the history of breast implants. Perhaps even more significant, however, are advances in the *non–device-related* process of breast augmentation itself, which have redefined the outcome and patient experience for this procedure.[1] These refinements in breast augmentation technique have been particularly salient for ensuring optimal use of form-stable breast implants.

Form-stable cohesive gel implants are a small subset of implants currently available in the United States, and they are available only through FDA premarket approval (PMA) clinical trials. There has been some confusion regarding what a cohesive gel implant actually is. Although all implant fillers are cohesive in the physical sense (whether saline or gel) the term *cohesive gel implant* has traditionally implied a form-stable device (e.g., Inamed 410, Mentor Contour Profile Gel [CPG]). Interestingly, even these devices are not truly form stable and exhibit different degrees of stability or cohesiveness in the various subgroups. These differences are cogent, because the benefits of form-stable implants that have been realized are a function of the form stability of the filler.

There is also no uniform opinion regarding the number of silicone implant generations that there have been. This is not the focus of this article, however, and in the end it is not truly important what generation an implant is. What is important are the device characteristics that ultimately impact soft tissue dynamics and patient outcomes.

Form-stable cohesive gel implants have been used internationally for longer than 10 years and have gained in popularity for aesthetic and reconstructive breast surgery. These implants may be available in the United States as soon as 2007 and will provide patients and surgeons with enhanced results if used properly. However, for most plastic surgeons in the United States there will need to be a transition from the technique used for smooth round saline implants to a more comprehensive approach.

ADVANTAGES AND DISADVANTAGES

When considering the advantages and disadvantages of current-generation cohesive gel devices it is important to keep in mind that they are directly related to the specific characteristics of each device as well as the physical condition of the patient. Therefore generalizations are not possible, because what is true for one specific device and patient

7

Advantages of Current-Generation Cohesive Gel Devices

- Long shell life
- Low risk of capsular contracture
- Less rippling than previous-generation devices
- Less soft-tissue stretch than previous-generation devices
- Cosmesis: Shape, maintenance of upper pole fill
- Safety
  - Minimizes negative effect of prosthesis on tissue
  - Less parenchymal atrophy than previous-generation devices
  - Less chance for traction rippling than previous-generation devices
  - Little gel migration if shell ruptures

may not be true for a different device. For example, rippling depends directly on the form stability of a device, which is determined by its degree of gel cohesiveness, the fill volume/mandrel volume ratio, gel-shell interaction, and the patient's skin quality. Hence, an implant that contains a firmer, more cohesive (more crosslinked) gel consistently produces very little rippling clinically (independent of patient soft tissue variables). An equally cogent point is that an implant that is more form stable and firm in one's hand will not necessarily be more firm or less natural in vivo. These types of misconceptions have no scientific basis.

Current data demonstrates increased longevity of the current-generation devices. The form stability of the filler results in less stress on the shell and in less folding, buckling, and wear over time. One study of 148 patients in Sweden who had 296 Style 410 implants placed during a 5- to 12-year period (mean follow-up 7 years) indicated that there were no clinical ruptures. However, MRI analysis revealed two ruptures (which were not confirmed or unconfirmed by surgical exploration) for a rupture rate of 0.6%, compared with 11.1% for earlier-generation, round gel devices.[2] Investigators from this same study describe these as lifetime devices.

Capsular contracture rates with the current form-stable devices have been low, likely because of two factors:

- The form-stable characteristics of the devices make them less compliant, which provides less mechanical advantage to a contracting capsule.
- These devices are typically associated with more refined surgical techniques that induce less tissue trauma and bleeding, which also impact capsule formation.[3]

Soft tissue stretch is not a fully controllable problem, but increased filler stability results in reduced stress on lower-pole soft tissue and likely less undesirable stretch over time.

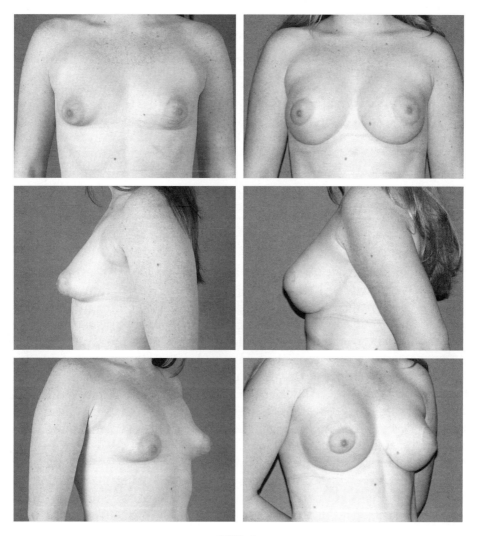

FIG. 1

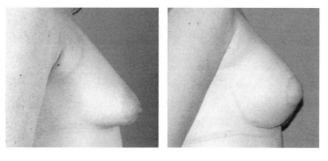

FIG. 2   **FIG. 3**

The ability of these new devices to favorably shape the breast is clinically evident as seen in this patient, who has excellent expansion and correction of a constricted lower pole. The breast has a different response to form-stable devices compared with earlier generations of gel and saline devices. The control of fill distribution within the breast is unparalleled, which allows for maintenance of upper pole fill over time that was not previously possible with other implants.

Disadvantages of Current-Generation Cohesive Gel Devices

- Require refined, meticulous process and technique
- Cost
- Require long incision that may limit certain approaches
- Firm
- Increased risk for rotation compared with round device
- Not appropriate for oversized requests
- Difficult secondary surgery

The safety benefits may turn out to be the most important aspect of these devices for patients. The known local effects of ruptured second-generation silicone implants have been well documented.[4] An exceedingly low rate of shell integrity loss in current-generation devices, coupled with the fact that the shell from these devices can be completely removed, and the filler will maintain its shape without migration, make many of the FDA's concerns about gel implant rupture irrelevant with the form-stable devices.

Disadvantages of cohesive gel implants include a requirement for more precise preoperative and intraoperative techniques (see box). This transition to a less familiar technique may make cohesive gel implants less appealing to some U.S. plastic surgeons. The costs of these devices are higher, incisions must be longer, and some approaches may be more difficult or not possible.

For the typical plastic surgeon in the United States, requests for a "Baywatch breast" by uneducated patients will not be effectively addressed using these devices, because oversized augmentations are not ideal. In the end, U.S. plastic surgeons will need to weigh the pros and cons of the devices; however, the additional benefits for patients will likely be the driving force for increased use of form-stable cohesive implants.

TECHNICAL CONSIDERATIONS

Form-stable cohesive gel devices need to be used with appropriate technique, but this is the case for any implant—recommended technique should always be followed. If the surgeon does not have good surgical control of the pocket (e.g., poor tissue, specific revision circumstances) these new devices are not recommended. Claims that these implants are too firm and do not move naturally have not been universally observed. However, the implant capsule appears likely to have more effect on both of these issues than does the degree of cohesion within the implant.

ESSENTIALS FOR SUCCESS

Success with current cohesive gel devices requires redefining how most U.S. plastic surgeons approach both aesthetic and reconstructive breast surgery. Although the current cohesive gel devices allow improved results, the real advances in breast augmentation are not about the implant. The techniques that have been used with success using these new devices will help minimize problems and optimize outcomes with any implant.

Breast augmentation is a process that includes the following important components[1]:
- Patient education and informed consent
- Tissue-based clinical planning
- Meticulous surgical technique
- Defined postoperative management

These four components should be performed consistently for every breast augmentation patient. When performed together they work synergistically to optimize outcomes. The goal is to maximize the quality outcome for the patient and minimize reoperation rates.

The data to support this process come from independently published series, peer-reviewed series, and series presented at national meetings, all indicating reoperation rates of 3% or less (compared with the standard 15%-24% from PMA studies over the past 15 years).[5-10]

Patient education is the most essential component of all, and patients should be given ample time using written material and patient educator sessions to define what their expectations are on paper. This is followed by a surgeon's consultation to reconcile the patients wishes with the reality of what is possible with their particular tissue configuration, allowing the patient to make final choices based on the comprehensive knowledge provided.

Tissue-based clinical planning is one large hurdle for plastic surgeons in the United States. A general reform from arbitrary and subjective implant selection and planning to logical, objective decisions based on tissue analysis will be required for successful implementation of the current cohesive gel devices. The high five planning process is a refinement of previous planning systems and allows surgeons to focus on the five critical decisions that determine outcomes in breast augmentation.[5] This system uses five measurements, the most important of which is the surgical base width of the breast, which is determined by taking the breast width minus the soft tissue thickness (Fig. 4). This

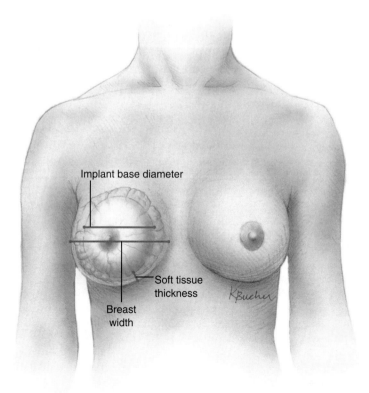

FIG. 4

planning process takes no longer than 5 minutes to perform, and it allows the surgeon to logically make all important decisions preoperatively regarding the following:

- Soft tissue coverage
- Implant volume
- Implant type
- IMF position
- Incision

The surgical technique is templated and systematic to minimize intraoperative decisions and maximize precise, atraumatic, bloodless dissection under direct vision. Creating a precise pocket to match the selected implant size is paramount.

Postoperative adjuncts (e.g., drains, pain pumps, narcotics, bras, straps, and restrictions) are minimized or eliminated, and specific postoperative instructions are given to allow the patient to return to normal activities within 24 hours and enhance the overall experience.

The four essential components of breast augmentation have proven efficacious with all implants, but they are required for successful implementation of the current generation of cohesive devices in the United States.

Using these devices for breast reconstruction facilitates the surgeon's ability to obtain symmetry because of the many different implant sizes available. Additionally, these implants exhibit less rippling under the thin soft tissues of reconstructed breasts. It is essential for surgeons to control the pocket during the initial phases of tissue expansion using precise, retroactive, expanded pocket-width planning to allow the subsequent use of these devices.

CONCLUSION

Currently the rest of the world has embraced form-stable cohesive gel devices, whereas the U.S. experience has been limited to FDA clinical trials. However, full approval of these devices is on the horizon. When that time comes, U.S. surgeons will be required to adopt a different approach to breast implant surgery to optimize results and allow implementation of these devices without significant problems. The potential for superior outcomes will drive surgeons to recognize the power of these new devices and acquire the necessary training to use them effectively.

REFERENCES

1. Adams WP Jr. The process of breast augmentation. Plast Reconstr Surg (submitted for publication).
2. Heden P. Experience with cohesive gel implants. Third Annual Matrix Course, Stockholm, June 2005.
3. Brown MH, Shenker R, Silver SA. Cohesive silicone gel breast implants in aesthetic and reconstructive breast surgery. Plast Reconstr Surg 116:768; discussion 780, 2005.
4. Bondurant S, Ernster V, Herdman R, eds, Committee on the Safety of Silicone Breast Implants Division of Health Promotion and Disease Prevention Institute of Medicine. Safety of Silicone Breast Implants. Washington, DC: National Academy Press, 1999.
5. Tebbetts JB, Adams WP Jr. Five critical decisions in breast augmentation using five measurements in 5 minutes: The high five decision support process. Plast Reconstr Surg 116:2005, 2005.
6. Tebbetts JB. Dual plane (DP) breast augmentation: Optimizing implant–soft tissue relationships in a wide range of breast types. Plast Reconstr Surg 107:1255, 2001.
7. Tebbetts JB. Achieving a predictable 24-hour return to normal activities after breast augmentation: Part II. Patient preparation, refined surgical techniques, and instrumentation. Plast Reconstr Surg 109:293, 2002.

8. Adams WP Jr, Rios JL, Smith SD. Enhancing patient outcomes in aesthetic and reconstructive breast surgery using triple antibiotic breast irrigation: Six-year prospective clinical study. Plast Reconstr Surg 117:30, 2006.

9. Bengtson B. Experience with 410 cohesive gel implants. Presented at the Annual Meeting of the American Society of Aesthetic Plastic Surgery, New Orleans, April 2005.

10. Jewell M. S8 breast educational course. Presented at the Annual Meeting of the American Society of Aesthetic Plastic Surgery, New Orleans, April 2005.

Editorial Commentary

Dr. Adams provides us with some very useful basic information about cohesive gel implants. The material is clearly presented and should be digested and stored in preparation for the implants becoming available in the United States. Certain areas are highlighted to produce precise pockets created by accurate and, hopefully, bloodless dissection. Precision is extremely important when using cohesive gel implants, because it greatly minimizes the possibility of unsatisfactory results, including asymmetries and a need for further intervention. Rereading this chapter will help emphasize this point and will stimulate surgeons to concentrate on precision of technique.

Ian T. Jackson, MD

Dr. Adams makes a salient point, separating factors attributable to the implant from those properly belonging to the surgeon. Thus, even though we now believe that we have a better implant, we still need to look at other factors. The concept of "form stability" requires some elucidation. To take things to the extreme, a rock or a concrete block is form stable, because at standard temperatures and pressures it deforms or flows imperceptibly to the human eye. But clearly these form-stable devices would make very poor implant materials. When we say an implant is form stable, what we really mean to say is that it is less likely to pool at the bottom of the pocket than an old-fashioned, syrupy, less-cohesive device. A form-stable device must still be deformable with pressure or movement; otherwise it would not fulfill its other obligations for the attainment of a good result. The underlying principle here is that there are degrees of stability, and some applications require a device that is more stiff whereas other applications require softer devices. For example, less-deformable devices will be superior in situations where an abnormal skin envelope requires specific pressure to be applied on the inside of the pocket to expand the skin where it is needed. Softer devices will better match postpartum women who have softer parenchyma so that the parenchyma-device interface will be less palpable. However, this does not decrease the requirement for a proper tissue cover. Thin tissue overlying a soft device is a recipe for rippling and a poor outcome. Once a surgeon has gained enough experience with these devices, it will be abundantly clear that how it feels coming out of the box will be an excellent indicator of how it will feel in situ. Firmer implants are firmer, and softer implants are softer. Interestingly, the only clinical study on the subject was published merely as a letter to the editor.[1]

The "generations" of breast implants are important insofar as they help doctors keep in mind what the probabilities are when they are seeing patients in the clinic. It makes no sense to keep breaking down the taxonomic categories into finer and finer slices that are of dubious value.

I respectfully disagree with Dr. Adams about whether devices that are firmer in the hand are firmer in situ. Rippling and firmness are definitely related. A rock-solid implant made of, well, rock, would not ripple; neither would it feel good to the touch. Firmer implants are less likely to ripple or wrinkle, but at the expense of feeling firmer. That is fine in a younger patient with firm parenchyma, but it may become an issue in the fatty breast. In the end, it is not just the surgeon but the patient who needs to make a decision about which is most important for her. Most doctors are aware that an implant with some moderate encapsulation will not have rippling, even if the capsule is thin. Pressure against the device is important to help maintain the shape of the device, and therefore the softest breasts with the thinnest capsules have the greatest chance of revealing underlying implant irregularities (rippling). Firmer implants will feel firmer in situ and will wrinkle less, period.

Dr. Adams quotes a surgeon who states that "these are lifetime devices." I do not think that Dr. Adams really believes this—in fact he and I agree that we should strongly resist the temptation to make statements that might mislead our patients into thinking that these devices last forever. All implants have a potential to fail, and all patients should be told that they are likely to require another operation in their lifetime. Telling patients that they have a lifetime device will only lead to disappointment in the long run.

Dr. Adams notes that these devices have a lower capsular contraction rate, and he attributes this to better surgical technique. Perhaps, but I don't think I became a better surgeon because of the technique I use with these devices. I had a low capsule rate with saline devices, and it became lower with the gel devices. I can't explain it, but this needs further investigation to see if it is a real phenomenon or merely wishful thinking on our part.

These cohesive gel devices are definitely built better than previous types, and if my wife, sister, or child needed a device, I would want them to choose one of these devices over any other type. However, it would be unrealistic to assume that these devices remove the possibility that material can escape from the gel matrix. Surgeons must be aware that nonreactive silicone oils are absorbed into the gel to make it soft, and, if the shell integrity is breeched, these moieties could equilibrate with the serous bath surrounding the device, although the total amount is extremely low. The risks we are talking about are orders of magnitude smaller than with the more liquid varieties of silicone, but we need to know that the shell still plays a pivotal role in separating the gel from the patient.

In Dr. Adams's discussion of the essentials for success, I think the most important criterion for success is refusal to operate on patients who are not good candidates. The worst cases I have seen should never have had augmentation in the first place. Until surgeons are willing to refuse cases, there will continue to be bad outcomes. With proper patient selection as outlined by Dr. Adams, and appropriate surgeon training, the incidence of poor or bad outcomes should be close to zero. There is no excuse for 15% reoperation rates. Reading between the lines of the FDA submissions, we can see that "patient request" is a common reason for reoperation. The common reasons for patient request are unsatisfactory size and unsatisfactory shape. Again, reading between the lines, it seems as though patients are sometimes dealing with poor shape outcomes because surgeons do not understand the dynamics of a Snoopy (or waterfall) breast or its opposite, the double bubble. These patients often have soft breasts, but not an aesthetic outcome, and therefore they rightly seek correction. These are rather predictable outcomes and can be avoided completely with appropriate training.

Claudio De Lorenzi, BA, MD

REFERENCE

1. van Loon J, Hage JJ, Woerdeman LA, et al. How soft are Soft Touch breast implants? Br J Plast Surg 57:176-177, 2004.

Anatomic Cohesive Gel Implants: Reshaping the Breast in Different Body Types

José Luis Martín del Yerro, MD

Augmentation mammaplasty is one of the most frequently requested aesthetic surgery procedures today. The introduction of anatomic cohesive gel implants represents a significant advance in cosmetic breast surgery that has altered the nature of this well-accepted operation and enhanced its potential for excellent aesthetic results. With these implants it is now clear that breast augmentation does more than alter breast size—it also has the ability to change breast shape and dimensions. By increasing the size of the breasts, we are also remodeling and reshaping them, and in most patients additional adjustments to the configuration of the inframammary fold or the relative position of the nipple-areola complex may be required.

The shape of the augmented breast depends largely on the shape of the implant used for enhancement. That is why anatomic implants, which have a well-defined, stable shape, make it possible to remodel the breast with greater precision and predictability. By using shaped implants we can recontour the breast, altering it to fit the individual needs of each patient. We can modify its width, change its lateral projection, and alter the projection of the upper or lower poles and the nipple-areola complex.

Despite their obvious benefits, anatomic implants present some challenges. They are more difficult to use than round implants and require more precise and meticulous surgical planning. There is little margin for error. The proper implant choice for each patient, along with careful preoperative marking and meticulous surgical technique, are essential to obtain good results. The learning curve for using these implants is steep; classic ways of thinking about breast size and implant choice do not apply. The focus has shifted from just enhancing breast size to producing a proportional breast shape that is balanced and in harmony with the torso. Thus augmentation mammaplasty requires an assessment of the breasts as well as the adjacent structures.

STANDARDS OF BREAST BEAUTY

As plastic surgeons we understand that the goal of plastic surgery is not to pursue perfection but to seek improvement. Aesthetics in breast surgery is a desirable but elusive goal. The patient's physical condition, the surgeon's skill, the operative approach selected, and the patient's expectations are all factors that influence the ultimate result. The challenge is to enhance the patient's appearance while approximating the ideals of beauty or harmony that are most suitable for that individual. Although the ideal is seldom present in nature, it is helpful to have a good understanding of breast aesthetics so that we have a standard of beauty to guide us in planning surgery.

Breasts are symmetrical structures found on the anterolateral walls of the thorax. Understanding the relations of the breasts to each other and to the torso is essential for evaluating the balance, proportion, and harmony of these structures. It is obvious that a morphologic analysis of breast beauty cannot be restricted to the breast itself, and that the torso and the rest of the body must also be analyzed. The breasts stand out and show their contour, beauty, and attractiveness against the backdrop of these other structures. The shape of an attractive or beautiful breast also depends on the proportions and shape of the torso. For educational purposes it is useful to compare the breast with the nose. The nose must maintain harmonious proportions within the face that frames it. In the same way that a large, thin, and pointed nose may spoil the harmony of a face with broad, flattened features, a breast with a narrow implantation base is unaesthetic on a broad, short torso.

Body Types and Breasts

The *breast implantation base* is the area of the thorax from which the breast mass projects. This area ranges from a few centimeters below the clavicle to the inframammary fold vertically and from a few centimeters from the sternal medial line to the anterior axillary line (or more laterally in some cases) horizontally.

Variations in body type produce variations in the breast implantation base, and the shape of this base may vary. In many cases it is circular; however, it may also be oval with a longer vertical axis or oval with a longer horizontal axis.

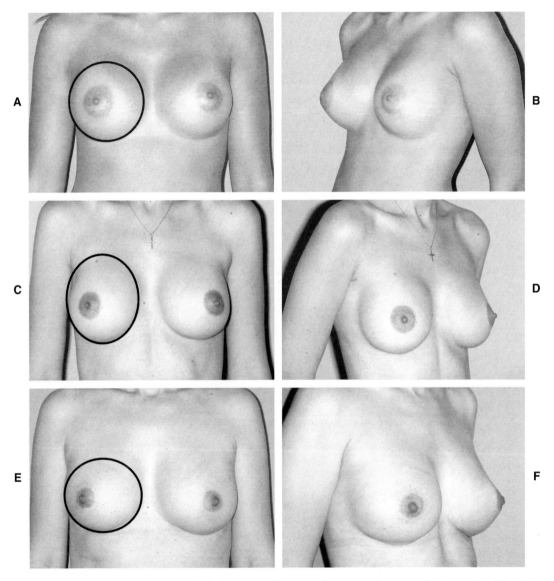

FIG. 1   Different possible shapes of the breast implantation base. **A** and **B,** Circular base. **C** and **D,** Oval base with larger vertical axis. **E** and **F,** Oval base with longer horizontal axis.

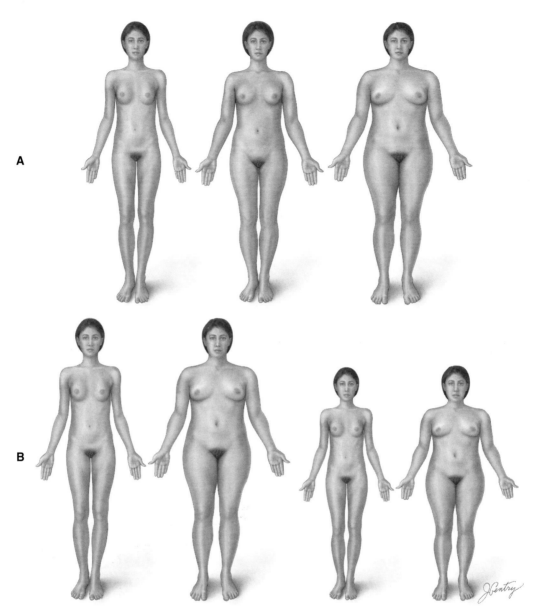

FIG. 2 A, The *asthenic* or *ectomorphic* body type corresponds to a thin body, lightly muscled and small shouldered *(left)*. The *pyknic* or *endomorpohic* body type corresponds to a thick body, heavily muscled and broad shouldered *(right)*. Between these is the *intermediate* body type *(center)*. **B,** The body type of any woman does not directly correlate to her height. Every body type can be found in both short and tall women.

The ratio between the width and height of the breast implantation base is not fixed in all women; it varies depending on the body type. A woman with an *asthenic* or *ectomorphic* body type—that is, someone who is thin, lightly muscled, and small shouldered—typically has breasts with vertical dimensions larger than the horizontal dimensions. A woman with a *pyknic* or *endomorphic* body type is thicker of body, heavily muscled, and broad shouldered; she should have breasts that occupy the entire width of the torso without being excessive in the vertical dimension. It is the body type, and especially the proportions, that determine the ratio between the height and width of the breast implant base, and not the absolute dimensions of the patient.

An asthenic body type can be tall or short, as can a pyknic body type. For an aesthetically pleasing result, the height/width ratio of the torso must be maintained in the implantation base of the new breast. The most common body type (in Caucasian women) is an intermediate one in which the height and width of the breast are similar, having an implantation base that is practically circular.

The Shape of the Breast

Because the height/width proportion of the breast implantation base varies, the shape of the breast also varies. It is helpful to first consider the ideal breast shape for a woman of an intermediate or "normal" body type and then consider the variations observed in other body types. Breast proportions and beauty standards are most effectively seen with the woman standing.

The Intermediate or "Normal" Body Type
Nipple-Areola Complex Position

The nipple-areola complex must be located over the point of maximum anterior projection of the mass of the breast.

The Upper Pole

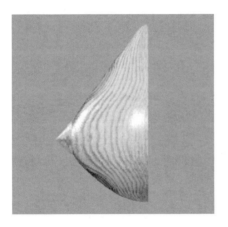

FIG. 3

The breast mass above the nipple-areola complex is called the *upper pole.* It starts a few centimeters below the clavicle and descends, following a gentle curve (slightly convex or straight) until it reaches the upper edge of the nipple-areola complex. It has a geometric form similar to half of a truncated cone.

The Lower Pole and the Inframammary Fold

The *lower pole* of the breast is located below the nipple-areola complex. It is similar in shape to a quarter sphere, but because the breast is situated on the curved plane of the thorax, the lateral portion extends along the side of the chest and is longer and larger than the medial portion.

The *inframammary fold* is the skin fold that defines the intersection between the lower edge of the breast and the skin of the abdomen. It is of particular importance for remodeling the breast and is the foundation that supports and defines the shape of the breast and its relation to the torso. It is truly from the inframammary fold upward that the rest of the breast is constructed.

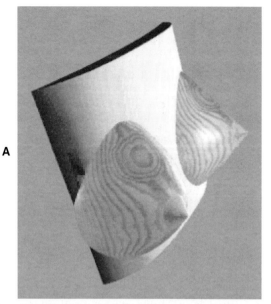

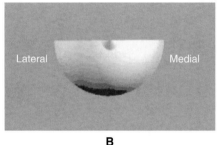
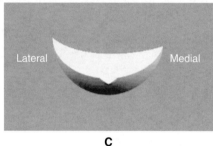
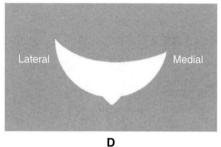

FIG. 4

Because the breast is located over the curved plane of the chest wall, the lateral portion of the breast serves to hold the nipple-areola complex in a relatively anterior position, causing the lateral portion of the lower pole to be larger in volume and area (see Fig. 4, *B* through *D*).

The 25-year-old woman shown in Fig. 5 presented with a tight skin envelope of low compliance. She had never been pregnant, nor had she lactated. Anatomic cohesive gel implants (11.5 cm wide, 10.8 cm high, 4 cm projection) were implanted in a pocket under the pectoralis major muscle using an incision in the inframammary fold. In the 1 year postoperative view, note that the new inframammary fold is not concentric with the nipple-areola complex; it extends further from it as it goes from medial to lateral. The incision is set precisely on the new inframammary fold.

When designing a new inframammary fold during augmentation mammaplasty, it must be remembered that the inframammary fold is not concentric with the nipple-areola complex, but rather moves away from it as it passes from the medial to the lateral areas.

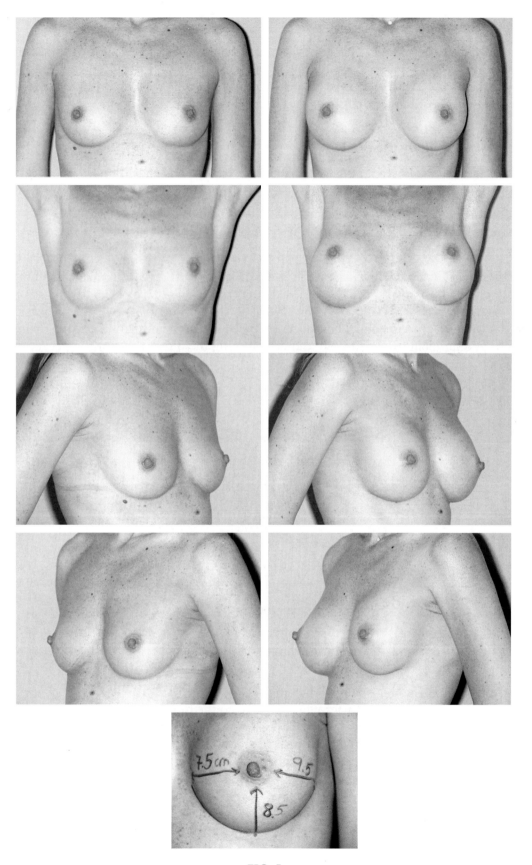

FIG. 5

The Pyknic Body Type

The differences between body types may affect the width/height ratio of the breast implantation base. In pyknic body types the implantation base is broader than it is tall, giving the breast a more flattened shape. Typically, these breasts have ample lateral extension, and the inframammary fold is not very low.

The Asthenic Body Type

In the asthenic body type the breast extends vertically. The chest is narrow compared with its height, and the same is true of the breast implantation base.

ANATOMIC EVALUATION OF THE PATIENT
Calculation of the Body Type

When surgically remodeling a breast, it is essential for the surgeon to take careful measurements of the patient's body and the existing breast. The shape of the new breast and its position on the torso will be planned based on these measurements. These measurements will also prove helpful when selecting the shape of the implant, marking the new inframammary fold before surgery, and determining the dimensions of the pocket that will hold the implant.

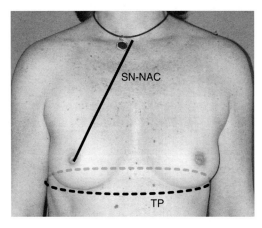

FIG. 6

These measurements include the following:
- Distance from the suprasternal notch (SN) to the nipple-areola complex (NAC): SN-NAC
- Thoracic perimeter at the level of the existing inframammary fold: TP
- Width of the breast to be remodeled

Once these measurements have been obtained, TP is divided by SN-NAC:

$$\frac{TP}{SN\text{-}NAC} = Y$$

The value Y is an indication of the ratio of the height and width of the torso in the area of the breast and therefore gives us, in an objective and quantifiable manner, the body type of the patient in relationship to the breast implantation base.

When this calculation is performed on a sufficient number of patients and the results are graphed, a Gaussian curve is obtained on which most are in a central position, with a Y value close to 4 (between 3.8 and 4.2), and two minima at the upper and lower ends.

When Y is greater than 4.3, the body type is pyknic and corresponds to women with proportions that are broader than they are tall. When the Y value is less than 3.7, the body type is asthenic, with long vertical lines. Patients between those two values have an intermediate body type.

There are no clearly defined boundaries between these body types. The transition from an asthenic to an intermediate body type, and from an intermediate to a pyknic body type, is a gradual one.

It is important to note that these calculations are reliable only in cases of mammary hypoplasia in which no ptosis or defects in mammary development have occurred. The calculation can still be applied when these conditions are present, but mastopexy or an appropriate correction must be planned simultaneously. In these cases we take the measurements in relation to the final position of the nipple-areola complex once the correction is made and not the measurements of the patient before the mastopexy.

PLANNING
Breast Shape and Dimension

In augmentation mammaplasty the lower pole of the breast receives the greatest remodeling. The upper pole of the breast and the nipple-areola complex project more over the chest wall, but this change requires little or no cutaneous expansion, which is why the nipple-areola complex is displaced upward during breast augmentation. However, the lower pole must undergo great change because this is where most of the volume is added, and therefore the area of the skin covering must be greatly increased. Note that remodeling a breast with an implant expanding and shaping its lower pole generally requires the creation of a new inframammary fold in a lower position.

Following the beauty standards we have described, the lower pole of the breast and the outline of the inframammary fold must be designed according to the patient's body type in an attempt to obtain results with the greatest possible harmony of proportions.

Selection of the Implant
Anatomic Implant

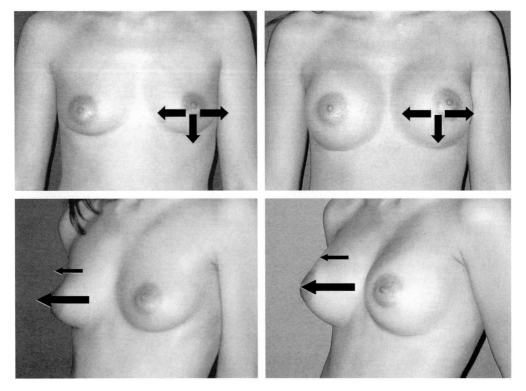

FIG. 7

In my opinion, anatomic implants permit improved reshaping of the breast in line with the aesthetic principles discussed here. They provide a stable, predictable means of breast enhancement. These implants reshape the lower pole without overfilling the upper pole, thus avoiding unnatural-looking results.

High-Cohesive Gel Implants

The high-cohesive gel implant has shape memory, allowing it to recover after deformation and remain stable over time. The shape does not depend on the covering of the implant; instead it is dependent on the gel itself. The gel allows the implant to be deformable and soft, with edges that are scarcely perceptible. These characteristics allow the surgeon to plan the shape of the new breast, estimating its dimensions very precisely.

Therefore, from a theoretical as well as a practical point of view, extracapsular rupture of the implant is not possible (no cases have been described in the literature); this is an enormous advantage over liquid gel or less cohesive implants in terms of safety, stability, and durability.

Implant Size

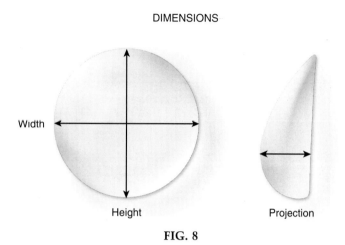

FIG. 8

The size of an implant must be considered in terms of its height, width, and projection and not its volume. The volume of the implant results from these other dimensions.

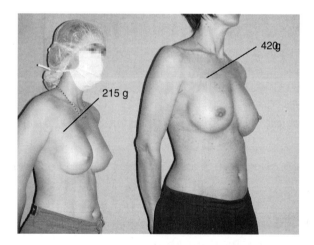

FIG. 9

The size of an implant is also related to size of the patient. Women with large frames require larger implants than women with small fames to achieve a balanced and harmonious appearance. We do not recommend maximum or minimum sizes, because what is disproportionate for one woman might be appropriate for another.

Implant Width

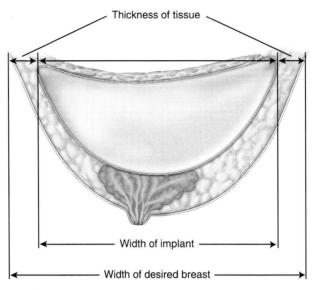

FIG. 10

The width of the breast is equal to the width of the implant plus the thickness of overlying tissues on each side.

$$\text{Width of desired breast} = \text{Width of implant} + (\text{Thickness of tissues} \times 2)$$

The thickness of the tissues is determined by a pinch test—the result of this test is already multiplied by two because the pinch encloses two layers. I determine the width of the desired breast by estimating the most medial and lateral points. This distance is measured with calipers.

The following formula makes it easy to determine the width of the implant and its value:

$$\text{Width of implant} = \text{Width of desired breast} - (\text{Thickness of tissues} \times 2)$$

This formula demonstrates that the width of the implant is calculated based on the width of the desired breast and the thickness of the tissues and assumes a fixed and objective value. Only these two parameters are used to select the width of the implant, which is independent of other measurements taken.

Implant Height

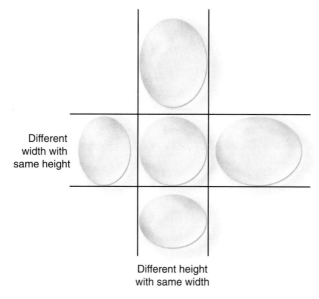

Different
width with
same height

Different height
with same width

FIG. 11

Although the width of the implant is a fixed and objective value, the height is a relative value. The height of the implant is related to its width. Currently a wide variety of implants with different shapes are available. Therefore if the height is varied for a given width, there are a number of options to choose from: implants with a circular base (where the height and width are equal), implants with a vertical oval base (where the width is less than the height), or implants with a horizontal oval base (where the width is greater than the height).

To determine the height of the implant to be used (with a circular, vertical oval, or horizontal oval base) the physician must look at the patient's body type and select the type of implant that will help remodel the breast to attain the most aesthetic appearance.

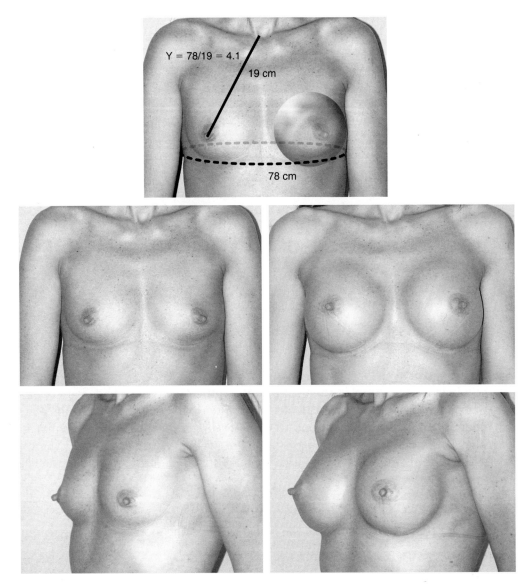

FIG. 12

Women with an intermediate habitus and a Y value close to 4 require an implant with a circular base.

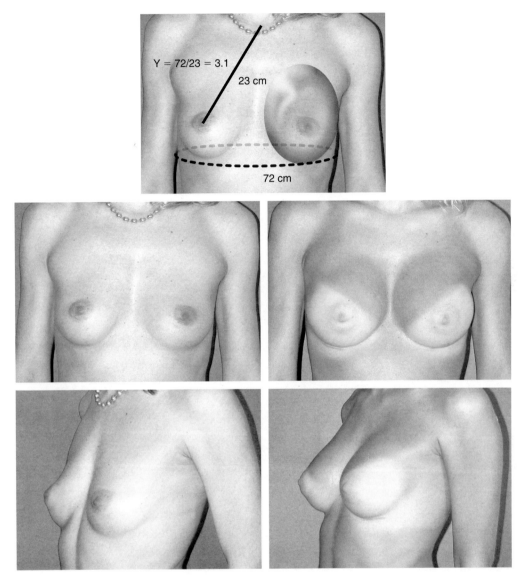

$Y = 72/23 = 3.1$

23 cm

72 cm

FIG. 13

Women with an asthenic body type and a Y value less than 3.7 require an implant with a base that is higher than it is wide (vertical oval). For example, this woman has an asthenic breast type; the TP is 72 cm and the SN-NAC distance is 23 cm. The Y value is 3.1; therefore the implant should have an oval base with a greater vertical axis to permit reshaping of the breast with good fill in the upper pole without causing a disproportion between the width of the breast and the torso.

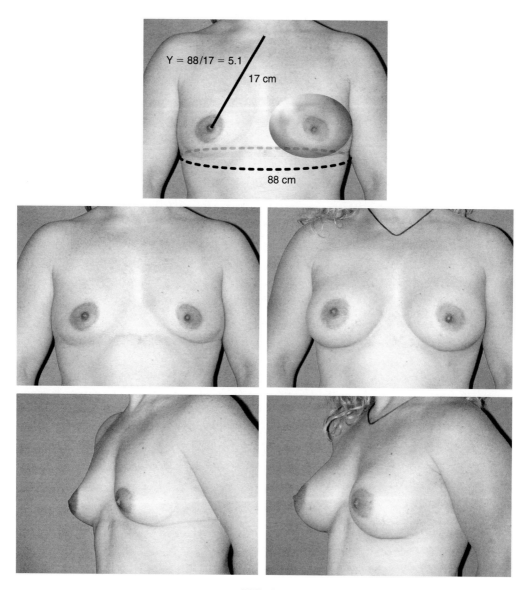

FIG. 14

On the other hand, for women with a pyknic body type and a Y value greater than 4.3, the implant must be wider than it is tall (horizontal oval). This woman has a TP of 88 cm and an SN-NAC distance of 17 cm. The Y value is 5.1, which is clearly a pyknic body type. An implant with an oval base having a longer horizontal axis was used for this patient.

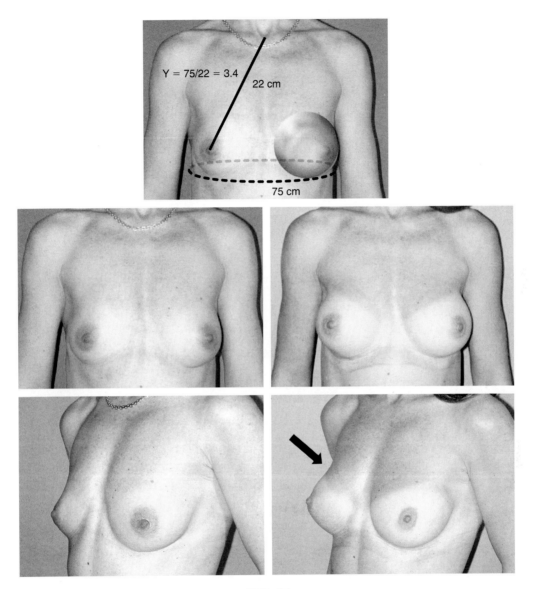

FIG. 15

For teaching purposes, let us consider a case in which the implant was poorly selected. This patient had a TP of 75 cm and the SN-NAC was 22 cm. The Y value was 3.4, so her body type was asthenic. An implant with an oval base having a larger vertical axis was indicated, but an implant with a circular base was actually used. The results are not optimal, with insufficient fill in the upper pole of the breast.

The boundaries between the various body types are not precise, and a gradual transition can be observed between the different body types. In these transitional cases, clinical judgment and discussions with the patient help the surgeon select an implant most suitable to each individual.

Implant Projection

The projection, or the anteroposterior dimension, of an implant must be determined using the patient's wishes and existing tissue. The patient's desire for a breast with greater or lesser projection will determine the implant profile chosen. If the patient prefers minimal or moderate augmentation, then an implant with low projection should be chosen. If greater enhancement is desired, implant projection must be increased accordingly.

It is important to note that existing tissues, their elasticity and thickness, quantitatively limit breast augmentation. The surgeon must estimate the projection of the implant that can be safely used and not exceed it, thereby producing natural, safe results that are stable over time.

Preoperative Marking

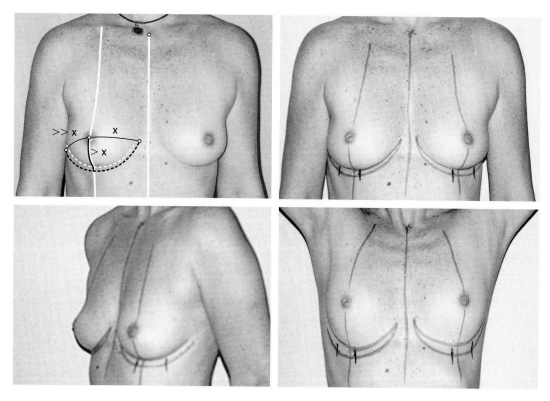

FIG. 16

Preoperative markings should be made on the patient's skin with colored markers, showing reference points and lines on the torso as well as the new inframammary fold and the position of the incision. The markings are made with the patient in an upright position immediately before the patient enters the operating room.

We start by drawing the anterior central line on the torso, followed by the preexisting inframammary fold and the medial line dividing the lateral and medial halves.

The most medial point of the breast to be reshaped (the desired breast) is then marked. The distance between these points on both breasts should not be less than 3.5 cm. The distance is measured from this point to the nipple, stretching the skin slightly. This measurement, which we call x, is the length of the medial pole once the implant has been inserted.

Next we mark the position of the new inframammary fold. In accordance with the canons of beauty described previously, the inframammary fold will not be concentric with the nipple. Laterally it will be further from the nipple-areola complex than it is in the medial portion.

In an intermediate body type, the most caudal point of the inframammary fold intersects the vertical axis of the breast, and its distance from the nipple is 2 to 5 mm longer than x (Fig. 16). When transferring this measurement to the lower pole the skin must be stretched, simulating the expansion effect of the implant when it is in place. The most lateral point of the new inframammary fold is determined by adding 5 to 10 mm to the x measurement.

When marking patients who have a pyknic or endomorphic body type, the most caudal point of the inframammary fold is more cranial than the canons of beauty indicate, and it should be marked at a distance nearly equal to x. In asthenic or ectomorphic body types this point should be marked more caudally by adding 5 to 10 mm to x.

Above all, it is important to understand that the inframammary fold is not concentric to the nipple-areola complex. In addition, the inferolateral quadrant should have a greater length and volume compared with the inferomedial quadrant, and these dimensions and relationships provide a more anterior orientation for the nipple-areola complex and a more natural, attractive lateral fullness for the breast.

Absolute measurements are not always recommended in surgery. Ultimately, all standards and measurements are subject to the clinical and artistic judgment of the surgeon. So understanding these concepts and applying these measurements with the subjective appreciation required by plastic surgery (a combination of science and art) is indispensable.

Finally, the incision is marked. It must be placed precisely over the new inframammary fold and be given a length of 5 cm: 4 cm lateral to the medial line of the breast and 1 cm medial to it. This is the part of the inframammary fold where the greatest amount of ptosis occurs and where the incision will be most easily concealed.

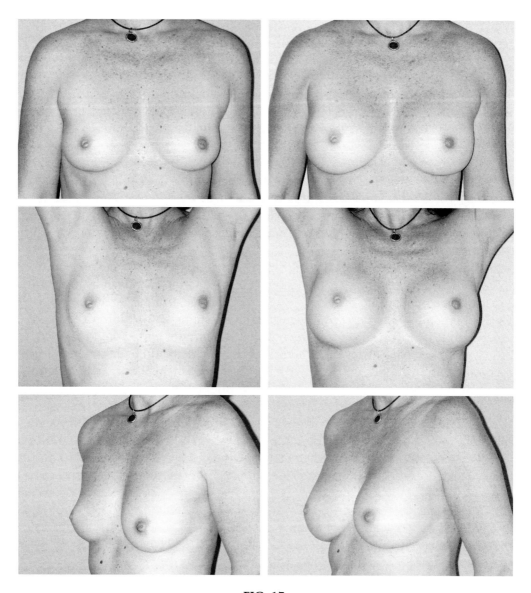

FIG. 17

This nulliparous 42-year-old woman presented with a skin envelope of mild compliance. Anatomic cohesive gel implants (12 cm wide, 11.3 cm high, 4.2 cm projection) were placed in subpectoral pockets. She is shown 1 year postoperative.

CONCLUSION

- Augmentation mammaplasty today should be viewed as a remodeling operation, performed to achieve an attractive breast shape and a harmonious relationship between the breast and the torso.
- Depending on the patient's body type, the shape of the breast and its implantation base on the thorax will vary. For women with an intermediate body type the implantation base is circular; for pyknic body types it is oval with a greater horizontal axis; for asthenic body types, the base is oval with a greater vertical axis.
- Anatomic implants permit surgeons to perform augmentation mammaplasty with greater predictability and harmony of proportions between the breast and the torso.
- The body type of a patient can be calculated simply, based on a few measurements. These measurements facilitate selection of the mammary prosthesis with the most appropriate implantation base for each patient.
- The transition between the intermediate body type and the other body types is not abrupt; there are many patients in the transitional zone for whom the surgeon's subjective appreciation and artistic gifts are key for selecting the right implant.
- Meticulous planning and preoperative marking are essential for achieving optimal results.

SUGGESTED READINGS

Angell M. Shattuch lecture evaluating the health risks of breast implants: The interplay of medical science, the law, and public opinion. N Engl J Med 334:1513-1518, 1996.

Heden P, Jernbeck J, Hober M. Breast augmentation with anatomical cohesive gel implants: The world's largest current experience. Clin Plast Surg 28:531, 2001.

Heitmann C, Schreckenberger C, Olbrisch RR. A silicone implant filled with cohesive gel: Advantages and disadvantages. Eur J Plast Surg 21:329-332, 1998.

Rohrich RJ, Beran SJ, Ingram AE Jr, et al. Development of alternative breast implant filler material: Criteria and horizons. Plast Reconstr Surg 98:552-560, 561-562, 1996.

Spear S. Breast augmentation with reduced height anatomic implants: The pros and cons. Clin Plast Surg 28:561-565, 2000.

Tebbetts JB, Tebbetts TB. The Best Breast: The Ultimate Discriminating Woman's Guide to Breast Augmentation. Dallas, CosmetXpertise, 1999.

Tebbetts JB. Dimensional Augmentation Mammaplasty Using the BioDimensional System. Santa Barbara, CA: McGhan Medical, 1994.

Tebbetts JB. Dual plane (DP) breast augmentation: Optimizing implant-soft-tissue relationships in a wide range of breast types. Plast Reconstr Surg 107:1255-1272, 2001.

Westreich M. Anthropomorphic breast measurement: Protocol and results in 50 women with aesthetically perfect breasts and clinical application. Plast Reconstr Surg 100:468-479, 1997.

Editorial Commentary

Dr. del Yerro emphasizes that when anatomic implants are used, it is very important to plan the shape and size of the implants. He cautions, quite rightly, that if an error in sizing is made, particularly if this is coupled with design, then an unfortunate result can occur. The prosthesis is stable when implanted, and if positioning is wrong, then the patient's natural breast will be unrelated to the underlying implant. As a result of that, a significant deformity can occur that is difficult to overcome. An additional, extremely significant feature is the patient's own anatomy. If this is disregarded, again the result will be suboptimal. Natural features such as the nipple/areolar complex position, the inframammary fold position, and the configuration of the fold are all important, and without paying attention to these the patient may be unhappy.

Another aspect that must be kept in mind is the width of the base of the breasts and how the implant must relate to this. Failure to take this into consideration will again end up with an unfortunate result.

A further aspect of cohesive gel implants is that various base shapes are offered that relate to the overall shape of the breast, which, in turn, is related to chest width and shape. Taking this into consideration is an important aspect of choosing the correct implant for the patient and, of course, ultimately achieving a satisfactory result.

It is the planning of the procedure that will give the best results. This is no longer the type of augmentation where one can place implants filled with saline or silicone gel and expect to have a satisfactory result. It is paramount that all aspects of the patient's breast and chest anatomy are carefully studied and assessed. With this information, an accurate implant size and shape can be estimated.

Ian T. Jackson, MD

Dr. del Yerro lucidly describes how breast shape necessarily follows anatomic constraints during development. Surgeons who wish to attain natural-looking results are advised to carefully study this article. Although he describes the location of the breast as beginning "a few cm below the clavicle," I advise surgeons to carefully study their collections of preoperative patient photographs. Patients generally do not have breast fullness above the line that crosses their chests transversely and connects the apexes of their anterior axillary folds. If surgeons carefully criticize their own postoperative results, any patient with fullness above this transverse line will look unnatural. I really like Dr. del Yerro's analysis of breast base shape, and his insights are excellent. I take several measurements similar to his, but I have not used the calculation of Y as described in the article, preferring to use my own methods developed over the years. Regardless of the technique used, the point is that individual surgeons are encouraged to use some form of objective method to determine these factors. The wonderful comparison drawings in this article bring to life the various shapes and shape relationships present in different body types. I predict that this article will be a classic of our generation, because even surgeons who do not use his measurements will gain insight into the basic shapes found in their patients. This can only help us to achieve better, natural-looking results. Keep these illustrations in mind when reading descriptions of shaped implants. Do the implants make sense from an anatomic standpoint? Will the breast tissue be supported properly in all orientations? Will there be excessive pressure on the tissues from these devices that will cause secondary changes and atrophy of the tissues? Surgeons must go beyond ad copy to understand the devices they are using and pressure manufacturers to provide what is required to achieve a "nondetectable" result that looks and feels like the real thing.

Claudio De Lorenzi, BA, MD

Characteristics of and Basic Technique for Cohesive Gel Implants

Claudio De Lorenzi, BA, MD

Cohesive gel anatomic implants offer decided advantages over traditional gel or saline implants for aesthetic and reconstructive breast surgery, producing stable, long-lasting breasts that are natural seeming and well contoured. However, these implants also require special care to ensure the best result. Basic decisions about implant shape, consistency, pocket size, and incision length are key to individualizing care and providing optimal results. Careful patient examination and effective patient education are also essential so that each patient understands the benefits and limitations of surgery and the special considerations necessary when these implants are used.

The technology exists to advance the art of augmentation mammaplasty to a new level with implants that are virtually undetectable. With careful patient selection and appropriate implant choice, we can in many cases get close to an ideal result that may be undetectable even by the patient's family physician. The goal is to predictably enlarge the breast while ensuring that it behaves like a natural, unaltered breast.

Different types of silicone implants are available outside the United States. Third-generation devices are still made with polydimethylsiloxane, but there is more cross-linking in them that gives them more characteristics of a solid by making the gel more cohesive. This gel may be deformed with compression and may be fractured if deformed beyond its limits. This is important, because if the surgeon tries to manipulate the device through an insufficient incision, it is possible to break the internal gel structure even though the external shell is intact, and the fractured gel may show through the skin as a deformity. This is a fundamental difference from previous generations of silicone devices, which had a fluid consistency. In addition, the shells of these devices have an intermediary barrier layer that prevents egress of short-chain molecules through the shell. I have used these devices since 2000 in more than 400 patients; patient satisfaction and breast appearance have been excellent.

PATIENT EVALUATION AND SELECTION

As with all breast surgery, a full medical history should be obtained, including any history of breast disease, breast cancer, and previous breast operations.

The physical examination provides important information to guide the surgeon in planning the procedure and selecting the appropriate implant. This examination should also be used as an opportunity to educate the patient about her appearance, to identify asymmetries, and to make certain that her expectations are realistic. It is helpful to show the patient what she looks like to others by taking an instant photograph of her chest/breast area while she is standing upright, arms at her side (Fig. 1). It is also helpful to draw directly on the photograph to point out any asymmetries of the inframammary fold, nipple height, or breast volume. During postoperative visits the marked photo will serve as a reminder to the patient of preexisting asymmetry. Asymmetries should be noted in the medical record.

The patient is examined while standing upright in front of the seated examiner. This is the most important part of the examination, because it allows the surgeon to assess the degree of breast ptosis and asymmetry. The patient should be examined with her arms in a number of positions: at her side, on her hips, and straight up. This last position will accentuate any asymmetry. These findings should be pointed out to the patient while she looks in a mirror. The patient is also examined in a bending position with her hands touching her knees to check her back for scoliosis, absent musculature, or other deformities that can sometimes relate to breast asymmetry.

The surgeon should assess the degree of skin laxity and the quality and quantity of soft tissue present to cover a proposed implant. Skin laxity can be assessed easily by asking the patient to assume the diver's position (Fig. 2) to demonstrate any lack of skin and soft tissue support. Patients with significant hanging skin should be advised that skin reduction (mastopexy) will also be necessary to achieve a good result. The patient's height and weight are recorded and specific measurements are made of the chest

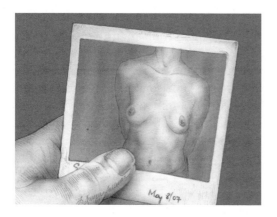

FIG. 1 Taking an instant photograph at the initial consultation helps patients identify issues more objectively than looking at themselves in a mirror. It also provides a record of the examination.

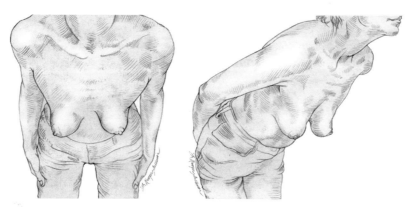

FIG. 2 The diver's position helps identify the degree of tissue laxity. Photographs of this position also help record the presence of preoperative loose skin.

(just under the axilla, over the bust), the breasts at maximum projection, the circumference of the chest at the height of the inframammary fold, the waist at the narrowest part, and the hips at the widest part. Measuring the interareolar distance, the distance to the nipple from the sternal notch, and the base width of each breast is also important. Careful records are kept of these measurements, and comparisons are made during follow-up visits.

An ideal patient will have a firm layer of subcutaneous fat, a sufficient amount of breast parenchyma, and excellent, thick skin with no striae cutis distensae (stretch marks). A less than ideal candidate will have very little subcutaneous fat, little natural breast parenchyma to hide the implant, and thin skin with innumerable striae cutis distensae.

CHOOSING AN IMPLANT

The choice of implant should be based on logical principles. For augmentation the goal is to enlarge the breasts without visible evidence of the underlying implants so that the breasts appear as natural as possible. All implants will be detectable to some degree. However, it is essential that the patient have sufficient soft tissue coverage so that the implant will not show through thin skin. Patients typically want full, natural-looking breasts, even if their physical attributes are not conducive to a good result. In any individual, larger implants will stretch the existing soft tissue envelope more than smaller implants. Consequently, larger implants tend to be more detectable.

As of this writing, all manufacturers are making implants so that the gel within each family of devices has the same degree of consistency, regardless of device size. This means that large implants are made with the same kind of gel used in small implants. Consequently, small devices appear somewhat stiff, and large devices tend to collapse under their own weight. In the future some manufacturers may alter the stiffness of their devices according to their size so that different sizes will behave in a similar fashion. In an ideal world, the gel at the base of each device would be stiffer to support the weight of the upper portion. In other words, the "degree of cohesion" of the silicone would vary not only between sizes (with larger sizes having more crosslinked material), but also within a single device so that the base could support the apex in an upright position.

Size

Implant size is an important consideration when selecting implants. Size is determined by the dimensions of the implant: the height, width, and projection. For most patients of average build, average-size implants with an average projection should be used. Good results can be obtained when these implants are used exclusively. Most experienced surgeons who have used implants over the years recall when only one size of implant was available. Good results were obtained with these devices, although more finesse is possible with tailored devices. Today, measurements play a far greater role in helping surgeons decide the volume and style of implant that is appropriate for each patient. Although a patient's wishes must be taken into consideration, the final implant volume selected will be determined primarily by what is appropriate for that patient's anatomy.

When selecting the appropriate implant size, several patient measurements need to be factored in. These include the patient's height, weight, chest diameter, base width of the natural breast, the degree of soft tissue laxity, and quantity of natural soft tissue (skin, fat, and parenchyma) that is available to hide the implant. How the patient is measured is important. The surgeon should choose a method and stick to it for consistently for all patients. In my practice I use a soft tape to measure the patient while she is standing in front of me. The width and thickness of the breast are important determinants of success. Calipers are positioned to measure the medial and lateral maximum extents of the breasts. If a breast is not well defined, then the nondominant hand compresses the breast to look for a line of demarcation showing its medial and lateral extent while the other hand holds the calipers.

If the breast shape is normal and the patient has an average body build, the breast width is used to determine implant size. A patient should have an implant selected based on the shape of her natural breast. For example, if the patient's natural breast width is approximately 9.5 cm in the upright position, it may not be a good idea to choose an implant wider than this (with some important exceptions for breast abnormalities). She would have to be counseled that "large implants" (which for her may include any implant wider than 9.5 cm) may cause undesirable outcomes. Because each manufacturer produces implants of different sizes, charts are provided to assist surgeons in the selection process. The charts are used during the consultation, and the measurement process is discussed in detail with the patient. The surgeon should caution the patient against making an inappropriate selection and inform her of potential undesirable consequences. Choosing an implant that is 15 cm at the base for the patient in the earlier example would result in inappropriate implant placement (too close together at the midline, or the meridian too far away from the natural midline, or the lateral aspects of the implant extending too far toward the midaxillary vertical, or a combination of all of these problems). Furthermore, this overlarge implant would stretch the patient's natural tissues, thinning them so that rippling of the implant shows through her skin. Sometimes these deformities will not occur for months or years after the surgery, appearing in conjunction with life events such as pregnancy, involution, and weight changes.

I find it helpful in my practice to keep some general numbers committed to memory to help calculate the anticipated increase in bra cup size related to the patient's weight (Table 1).

This table approximates the implant volume needed to obtain an approximate increase of one bra cup size. Total accuracy is not possible, because all bra manufacturers have different standard cup sizes. U.S. brands typically underestimate actual cup size, whereas European bras overestimate bra size, so that a woman can be an A cup and a C cup at the same time. Therefore these figures must be used only as a general guide.

An average patient in my practice is 5 feet, 6 inches tall, weighs 125 pounds, and has a single cup size of about 200 cc. In a smaller patient (e.g., 100 pounds), one cup size is approximately 150 cc. Similarly, a woman weighing more than 150 pounds may need approximately 250 cc to produce an increase of approximately one cup size (see Table 1). It is important for the physician to recognize that most patients want a bra size increase of about 1 or 1½ cups, and that the desired volume increase will vary with a patient's actual size. Returning to the example, if a petite 100-pound woman wants about one cup size of enlargement and she has good soft tissues with no ptosis and good skin, using a manufacturer's chart to look up her breast base diameter of 9.5 cm shows that a medium-height, 9.5 cm wide implant is 135 cc.

I usually choose implants from the medium height category unless special circumstances are present. If a patient is unusually tall (nearer to 6 feet), taller implants may be appropriate. On the other hand, shorter patients (less than 5 feet tall) may consider low height implants. In general, moderate height, moderate projection implants should be used. However, as the surgeon gains experience, finesse may be attained with other available sizes (Tables 2 through 11).

TABLE 1   Relationship of Patient's Weight to Implant Volume

Approximate Weight of Patient (lb)	Approximate Volume of Implant Needed to Increase by One Bra Cup Size (cc)
100	150
125	200
150	250

TABLE 2   Mentor Contour Profile Gel™ 312 and Mentor Cohesive III™, Low Height/Moderate Plus Profile

Volume (cc)	Width (cm)	Height (cm)	Projection (cm)
125	9.0	8.0	3.8
145	9.5	8.4	4.0
170	10.0	8.8	4.2
195	10.5	9.3	4.4
225	11.0	9.7	4.7
255	11.5	10.2	4.9
290	12.0	10.6	5.1
330	12.5	11.1	5.3
370	13.0	11.5	5.5
415	13.5	12.0	5.7
465	14.0	12.4	5.9
515	14.5	12.8	6.1
570	15.0	13.3	6.3
690	16.0	14.2	6.8

TABLE 3   INAMED Style 410LF Anatomic Cohesive Gel and Soft Touch Gel, Low Height/Full Projection

BioDIMENSIONAL™ Cohesive Gel-Filled Breast Implant With BIOCELL™ Surface Texture			
Implant Weight (g)	Width (cm)	Height (cm)	Projection (cm)
125	9.5	7.6	3.7
150	10.0	8.1	4.0
175	10.5	8.6	4.2
205	11.0	9.1	4.4
240	11.5	9.6	4.6
270	12.0	10.1	4.8
310	12.5	10.5	5.1
390	13.5	11.4	5.3
440	14.0	11.8	5.6
490	14.5	12.2	5.8
540	15.0	12.6	6.1
595	15.5	13.0	6.2

TABLE 4   Mentor Contour Profile Gel™ 321 and Mentor Cohesive III™, Medium Height/Moderate Profile

Volume (cc)	Width (cm)	Height (cm)	Projection (cm)
120	9.0	8.5	3.3
135	9.5	8.9	3.5
155	10.0	9.4	3.7
180	10.5	9.9	3.8
215	11.0	10.3	3.9
245	11.5	10.8	4.0
280	12.0	11.3	4.2
315	12.5	11.8	4.4
355	13.0	12.2	4.6
395	13.5	12.7	4.7
440	14.0	13.2	4.9
480	14.5	13.6	5.0
530	15.0	14.1	5.2
640	16.0	15.0	5.6
775	17.0	16.0	5.9

TABLE 5   INAMED Style 410MM Anatomic Cohesive Gel and Soft Touch Gel, Moderate Height/Moderate Projection

BioDIMENSIONAL Cohesive Gel-Filled Breast Implant BIOCELL Textured INTRASHIEL Barrier Shell Anatomic Shape			
Implant Weight (g)	Width (cm)	Height (cm)	Projection (cm)
160	10.0	9.1	3.6
185	10.5	9.6	3.8
215	11.0	10.1	4.0
245	11.5	10.6	4.2
280	12.0	11.1	4.4
320	12.5	11.6	4.6
360	13.0	12.1	4.8
400	13.5	12.5	5.0
450	14.0	12.9	5.2

If a patient desires a larger-volume device, then the surgeon may choose the same width implant with a higher projection. Thus the patient may satisfy her desire for a larger implant while the surgeon stays within the width restriction of her natural breast. For example, if we search for a 12 cm width device using Table 4, we find the volume of the device is 280 cc, and looking for the 12 cm width device using the medium height/ moderate profile in Table 6, we see the volume of the device is 330 cc.

What does one do if a patient has an abnormal breast? I generally avoid damaging the inframammary fold unless it is abnormal because, as those who have tried to create a new inframammary fold know, it is difficult. However, if a patient has a congenital anomaly that makes the inframammary fold abnormal, then it must be altered. In this case the rule of not using implants wider than the natural breast may not hold. These patients require measurements of their chest and an estimate of the breast base appropriate for their chest circumference. If the skin is of good quality, then I recommend placing the implant above the muscle so that the implant may exert force on the contracted skin to allow it to expand.

TABLE 6   Mentor Contour Profile Gel™ 322 and Mentor Cohesive III™,
Medium Height/Moderate Plus Profile

Volume (cc)	Width (cm)	Height (cm)	Projection (cm)
140	9.0	8.5	3.8
165	9.5	8.9	4.0
195	10.0	9.4	4.2
225	10.5	9.9	4.4
255	11.0	10.3	4.7
295	11.5	10.8	4.9
330	12.0	11.3	5.1
375	12.5	11.8	5.3
420	13.0	12.2	5.5
475	13.5	12.7	5.7
525	14.0	13.2	5.9
585	14.5	13.6	6.1
650	15.0	14.1	6.3

TABLE 7   INAMED Style 410MF, Moderate Height/Full Projection

Volume (cc)	Width (cm)	Height (cm)	Projection (cm)
140	9.5	8.6	3.7
165	10.0	9.1	4.0
195	10.5	9.6	4.2
225	11.0	10.1	4.4
255	11.5	10.6	4.6
295	12.0	11.1	4.8
335	12.5	11.6	5.1
375	13.0	12.1	5.2
420	13.5	12.5	5.3
470	14.0	12.9	5.6
525	14.5	13.2	5.8
580	15.0	13.6	6.1
640	15.5	13.9	6.2

TABLE 8   Mentor Contour Profile Gel™ 322 and Mentor Cohesive III™,
Medium Height/Moderate Plus Profile

Volume (cc)	Width (cm)	Height (cm)	Projection (cm)
165	9.0	8.5	4.6
195	9.5	8.9	4.8
225	10.0	9.4	5.1
260	10.5	9.9	5.3
300	11.0	10.3	5.6
345	11.5	10.8	5.8
390	12.0	11.3	6.0
440	12.5	11.8	6.2
495	13.0	12.2	6.5
555	13.5	12.7	6.7
620	14.0	13.2	6.9
685	14.5	13.6	7.1

TABLE 9   INAMED Style 410MX, Moderate Height/Extra-Full Projection

Volume (cc)	Width (cm)	Height (cm)	Projection (cm)
165	9.5	8.6	4.6
195	10.0	9.1	4.9
225	10.5	9.6	5.1
255	11.0	10.1	5.3
290	11.5	10.6	5.5
325	12.0	11.1	5.7
370	12.5	11.6	6.0
410	13.0	12.1	6.1
445	13.5	12.5	6.2
520	14.0	12.9	6.5
550	14.5	13.2	6.7
620	15.0	13.6	7.0
685	15.5	13.9	7.1

TABLE 10   Mentor Contour Profile Gel™ 322 and Mentor Cohesive III™, Tall Height/Moderate Plus Profile

Volume (cc)	Width (cm)	Height (cm)	Projection (cm)
145	9.0	9.4	3.8
175	9.5	9.9	4.0
205	10.0	10.4	4.2
235	10.5	10.9	4.4
270	11.0	11.5	4.7
305	11.5	12.0	4.9
350	12.0	12.5	5.1
395	12.5	13.0	5.3
445	13.0	13.5	5.5
495	13.5	14.1	5.7
555	14.0	14.6	5.9
615	14.5	15.1	6.1
680	15.0	15.6	6.3

TABLE 11   INAMED Style 410FF Anatomic Cohesive Gel and Soft Touch Gel, Full Height/Full Projection

BioDIMENSIONAL Cohesive Gel-Filled Breast Implant			
BIOCELL Textured INTRASHIEL Barrier Shell Anatomic Shape			
Implant Weight (g)	Width (cm)	Height (cm)	Projection (cm)
160	9.5	10.0	3.7
185	10.0	10.5	4.0
220	10.5	11.0	4.2
255	11.0	11.5	4.4
290	11.5	12.0	4.6
335	12.0	12.5	4.8
425	13.0	13.5	5.2
475	13.5	14.0	5.3
535	14.0	14.5	5.6
595	14.5	15.0	5.8
655	15.0	15.5	6.1
740	15.5	16.0	6.2

Consistency and Rippling

Different manufacturers use different cohesive gel consistencies in their breast implants. For example, Mentor's Contour Profile Gel (CPG) implant is similar in consistency to Inamed's Soft Touch devices. The Inamed 410 implant is firmer than the CPG. In my practice, there is a role for each type of implant; I try to match the texture of the patients' natural tissues with the texture of the implant. Most of my patients are postpartum, and if they have sufficient natural breast tissue then I typically choose either a Mentor CPG or an Inamed Soft Touch product for them because they are softer and "bouncier" in situ than the Inamed 410 device. If a patient has firmer breasts, I may recommend the regular Inamed 410 implant. Both the Mentor and the Inamed implants have desirable properties. The regular Inamed 410 is firmer, but it is also less likely to show rippling. Neither product has totally solved the rippling problem because it is mainly a patient selection issue. I have seen rippling with each of these devices. Most of the time rippling is position dependant, and the diver's position is excellent for demonstrating problems when they occur (see Fig. 2). If the physician opts for more firmness, the breasts will look less realistic when the patient is moving, walking, or lying down. However, if the physician opts for a softer, more natural feel, then slightly more rippling may occur. All of the devices are very well made, and patients should have a role in the decision process. I typically show patients samples of each device, discuss the benefits of each, and ask them to help choose the ideal device for them.

Patients with a thinner skin covering will have a greater tendency to show undesirable implant characteristics. This can be partly controlled by the surgeon who recommends the implant size. Larger sizes will distribute the same amount of tissue over a larger geographic volume, thereby resulting in a relative thinning of tissues—the larger the implant, the greater the problem. It is important to remember that living tissues respond to stresses, and that tissue expansion occurs with any implant. Both recruitment and new skin growth are to be expected with tissue expanders, so there will always be some extra skin over time in patients with implants.

The normal human breast is not static. Most women undergo biologic changes from puberty through adulthood, including maternity, lactation, and involution. The breast shape is not stable during these stages, and therefore an implant will have different appearances during the different stages. As they age, most women experience a natural loss of volume, especially in the upper part of the breast, in association with some de-

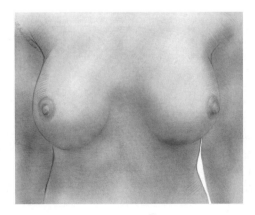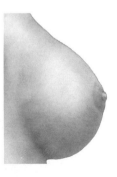

FIG. 3   With time, saline implants may show abnormalities along the periphery of the implant that are fill-volume and position dependent. These defects are rarely seen with cohesive gel implants.

gree of glandular ptosis. It is essential that women understand that if an implant is placed deep to the pectoralis muscle, then a waterfall or Snoopy deformity may eventually develop, because the parenchyma eventually drops below the implant that is supported by the muscle. Remember that breasts will eventually descend if there is significant parenchyma, whereas the chest muscles will not descend.

Surface Texture/Tissue Adherence

There is a common misconception that textured implants of a particular type always result in tissue ingrowth. Clinically, this has not been found to be the case. Typically, textured silicone gel-filled implants do not induce tissue ingrowth, regardless of the nature of the texture. Malrotation may occur with any type of shaped implant. The only exception to this is when great internal pressure is applied, such as with tissue expansion or tight submuscular pockets. Tissue expansion with textured devices can produce Velcro-like tissue adherence. I have had the opportunity to remove capsules of both moderately and aggressively textured implants during submammary augmentations, and in no case of normal breast augmentation was tissue ingrowth attained (in contrast with tissue expanders, in which the more-aggressive Inamed Biocell [salt loss] texture usually causes ingrowth, but the Mentor Siltex texture does not).

Most of the implants I place are in the subfascial space, not the subpectoral space. Therefore I prefer textured devices because they seem to have a lower rate of encapsulation when used in this area. There does not seem to be a clinical benefit to placing textured implants underneath the pectoralis, so in the event that submuscular placement is desired, smooth-walled implants would likely be successful. However, there is no hard and fast rule, and some surgeons use one type of implant exclusively.

BASIC TECHNIQUE
Markings

Planned incisions are marked with the patient standing. Because of the underlying Scarpa's fascia that extends onto the chest, the patient's arm position directly affects breast position. Therefore, markings on the patient's chest should be made with her arms in the same position that will be used on the operating table. If the patient were to be marked in the resting position (with her arms at her side), and then positioned on the operating table with arms abducted, the marks would be too high (Fig. 4).

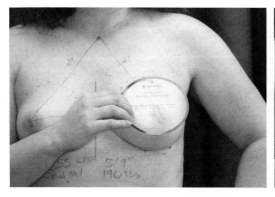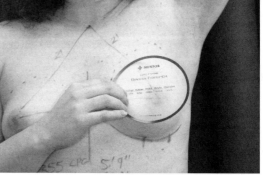

FIG. 4   The position of the upper line shows the pocket plan if the patient is marked in the anatomic position and then switched to the 90-degree, arm-abducted position on the operating room table.

Surgical Approach

The most common approaches used for cohesive gel implants are the periareolar and inframammary approaches because they afford the greatest flexibility and visibility for proper implant positioning (see p. 75 and p. 91 for these approaches). I personally prefer incisions on the breast. The scars are typically very good in the periareolar or inframammary regions, the incisions may be used again, and they do not require abnormal stresses to be applied to the gel implants during insertion. It is important to remember that cohesive gel implants may fracture, and that the firmer gels are more fragile. Colleagues who have used the axillary approach do not advise using it for the larger implant sizes that are typically used in North America.

Length of Incision

Unlike saline implants, which may be inserted empty and filled in situ, gel implants are fully formed. Therefore they require a larger incision for insertion. For typical 250 cc sizes, a 5 cm incision is sufficient, but larger incisions may be necessary for larger devices to avoid possible damage to the implant. Stiffer devices also need larger openings.

Implant Position

The submammary location, in which the implant is placed above the muscles, is less likely to show dynamic deformity with muscular activity, but it is also less likely to support a heavy breast implant and is therefore more prone to breast ptosis than the subpectoral or fully submuscular positions. The submuscular location is chosen for patients with very poor tissues who have little breast parenchyma and no excess skin. For submuscular placement, the pectoralis major muscle and portions of the serratus anterior muscle are elevated, and the implant is placed deep to the muscles, creating a complete submuscular and subfascial pocket. This is a moderately fast dissection, staying close to the rib periosteum. Extreme care must be exercised to avoid lowering the inframammary fold, using the rib subjacent to the inframammary fold as a handy reference point. If the patient has any degree of glandular ptosis, then maneuvers beyond the scope of this discussion are required to achieve success.

If the upper part of the breast at the proposed height of the implant is thin, much less than 2 cm, then a subpectoral position is appropriate. This is an effective method for reducing upper pole implant visibility, but it has a trade-off with a potential for abnormal breast dynamics. If the tissues are thin, the implant is positioned under the pectoralis where it will be far less likely to be visible. This is the easiest and fastest plane of dissection of the three presented. Dissection of the lower border of the pectoralis from the chest wall as well as from the breast may be required to allow the device to sit at the appropriate level on the chest wall. A firmer implant may be a better choice if this position is chosen because it will better resist deformation from muscular contraction. If the patient has 2.5 cm or more of firm parenchymal tissue across the superior (cephalad) region of her breast, then the Mentor CPG produces excellent results, especially in the subfascial position, effectively achieving a nondetectable result.

Plane of Dissection in a Submammary Procedure

The plane of dissection is critical when an implant is placed in the submammary position.[1-4] The plane of dissection should be subfascial, especially at the periphery of the pocket (Fig. 5). There are vertical and vascularized extensions of fascia that extend into the substance of the pectoralis muscle from the overlying fascia. This vascular plane cannot be dissected bluntly; good lighting and careful hemostasis through fulguration of bleeding vessels is important. Dividing these fibers allows elevation of the fascia. At the end of the subfascial dissection the muscle edge is tented up at the border of the implant pocket so that implant edge visibility is minimized[1] (see Fig. 5). The fascia itself may be quite thin and friable in some patients, particularly in the inferior pole, but it is usually thicker in the upper pocket area over the pectoralis major muscle and laterally over the serratus anterior muscle. The surgeon should dissect under the fascia at least 1 to 2 inches proximal to the edge of the implant pocket. I typically dissect a complete subfascial pocket, but it is often necessary to split the fascia under the central area to allow the implant to fill the central portion of the empty breast to create projection. I sometimes elevate the fascia at the periphery of the implant, leaving some of the central fascia intact on the pectoralis. This technique permits better camouflage of the implant edge and also reduces operating time because the central portion of the pocket can be developed more quickly above the fascial plane.

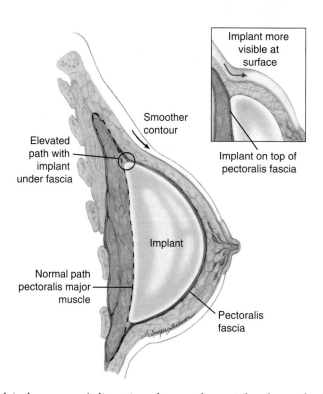

FIG. 5   Subfascial (submammary) dissection elevates the peripheral muscle tissue at the implant edge, resulting in better camouflage of the implant edge. It may also provide mild compression of the implant, which may better help to hold its shape.

Implant Pocket Size and Shape

When working with saline implants the pocket must be larger than the implant to promote softness by allowing the implant to move around in an oversized pocket. This is not true for cohesive gel implants. The pocket need only be large enough for the implant when the implant is compressed. Creating an oversized pocket for shaped implants introduces a greater risk of malposition.

The pocket shape must conform to the overall dimensions of the selected implant. For example, if the implant is wider than it is tall, then the pocket should also be wider than it is tall, otherwise the forces applied to the implant will cause it to turn sideways. Abnormally shaped implant pockets encourage implant malrotation and should be avoided.[2,5-8]

Drains may be required in some patients. I typically only use them when I have performed extensive dissections using electrosurgery because this could reasonably be expected to cause more serous effusions. For example, after capsulectomy, or if there are a very large number of bleeding vessels that required electrocautery, then I use a small suction drain brought out through a small axillary puncture wound. These should always be placed before implant insertion. I do not believe that drains prevent hematomas, but they may help prevent malrotation in some cases.

Implant Insertion

An assistant retracts the incision open while the surgeon places the implant in position. Anatomically shaped implants must be placed appropriately into the pocket. Using a clock reference, with 12 o'clock at the cephalic end of the implant and 6 o'clock at the caudal end, then typically the edge of the implant at 9 o'clock is placed against the left side of the incision. Then using the right index finger, the surgeon gently pushes the implant through the opening and stabilizes it with the nondominant hand. External compression of the implant gradually shifts most of the gel material from outside the pocket to inside the pocket until the implant has totally passed through the opening. Care must be taken not to deform these implants beyond their limits because the gel within the implant may fracture, even when the implant is intact externally. Implants that have been damaged when inserted often reveal surface irregularities through the breast tissue. It takes some practice to learn how much force is too much. Sample implants are useful to inexperienced surgeons for learning the limits of the forces that may be applied. Clinically the potential for fracture is greater with the firmer, more cohesive implants. There is no remedy for a fractured implant; it must be replaced.

Postoperative Management

Postoperatively it is prudent to apply a light dressing and support with a mildly adhesive porous tape. This will help hold the tissues in place. Patients should be advised to curtail their activities for the first few days and gradually increase activity as tolerated. Patients may shower on the day after surgery. Patients return for follow-up visits at 1 week, 4 weeks, 4 months, 12 months, and then annually thereafter. In addition, patients are encouraged to call the office to speak to the head nurse if they have any concerns. We record all measurements on standardized data sheets that are entered into a computer spreadsheet.

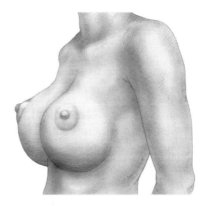

FIG. 6   Excessive release of the inframammary fold often results in a bottoming-out deformity.

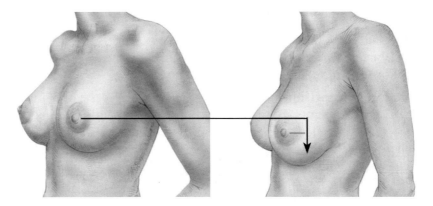

FIG. 7   Gravity pulls more on larger breasts, eventually resulting in ptosis. Larger implants will cause more skin stretch and more descent with time, especially in the submammary position.

PREVENTABLE PROBLEMS

If the inframammary fold is not respected during the procedure, several problems may occur. If the inframammary fold is released completely during the submammary dissection, the breast implant may descend precipitously, resulting in an abnormally high nipple position on the resulting breast mound. This has sometimes been called *bottoming out* (Fig. 6). In my opinion this problem is iatrogenic because it can be prevented by not altering the inframammary fold unless it is affected by pathology, as in the case of a constricted breast. Because of their weight, all implants exert a downward force that will alter tissue characteristics over time. Thus the breast will descend on the chest wall, mimicking the natural process of breast ptosis (Fig. 7). The patient should be informed that breast ptosis is a natural consequence of large breasts, and this should be a consideration when choosing breast implant size. Other preventable problems include the Snoopy or waterfall deformity and the double-bubble deformity (Fig. 8).

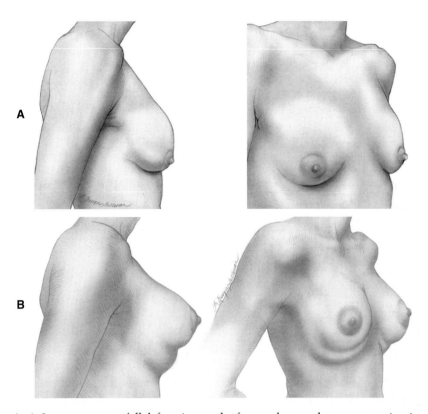

FIG. 8   A, A *Snoopy* or *waterfall* deformity results from submuscular augmentation in patients with glandular ptosis because the implant location prevents redistribution of glandular tissue. Correction requires either an aggressive mastopexy or, if glandular tissue conditions permit, a device exchange to a cohesive gel product and a site exchange to a subglandular position. **B,** A *double-bubble* deformity occurs when an implant has been placed subpectorally and the inframammary fold has been released but the glandular attachments to the pectoralis have not been released. Correction is performed by releasing the fascial connections between the lower border of the pectoralis major muscle and the breast and by separating the gland from the skin. Sometimes radial glandular incisions are also required to redistribute the glandular tissue. This deformity typically occurs in constricted breasts.

CONCLUSION

Each surgeon must maximize the chances of success with cohesive gel implants by carefully following the correct paradigm. For surgeons who have not had experience using these devices, it would be helpful for them to educate themselves about the properties of and special considerations for using cohesive gel implants. Measurements are the key to success with these devices. We should always measure each patient and record these measurements, if only to elevate the science of the work we do. Counseling patients is time-consuming but rewarding, and it helps avoid postoperative misunderstandings. The surgeon who spends time educating the patient should have better outcomes and better patient follow-up. Long-term follow-up is essential because if we only saw 6-week results, we would think that nothing ever went wrong with augmentation surgery. However, the early result is never really the final result. Following patients carefully over many years will teach us more than could ever be taught during residency, and it helps us become better surgeons.

REFERENCES

1. Góes JC, Landecker A. Optimizing outcomes in breast augmentation: Seven years of experience with the subfascial plane. Aesthetic Plast Surg 27:178-184, 2003.
2. Graf RM, Bernardes A, Rippel R, et al. Subfascial endoscopic transaxillary augmentation mammaplasty. Aesthetic Plast Surg 24:216-220, 2000.
3. Graf RM, Bernardes A, Auersvald A, Damasio RC. Subfascial breast implant: A new procedure. Plast Reconstr Surg 111:904-908, 2003.
4. Barnett A. Transaxillary subpectoral augmentation in the ptotic breast: Augmentation by disruption of the extended pectoral fascia and parenchymal sweep. Plast Reconstr Surg 86:76-83, 1990.
5. Spear SL. Breast augmentation with reduced-height anatomic implants: The pros and cons. Clin Plast Surg 28:561-565, 2001.
6. Heden P, Jernbeck J, Hober M. Breast augmentation with anatomical cohesive gel implants: The world's largest current experience. Clin Plast Surg 28:531-552, 2001.
7. Baeke JL. Breast deformity caused by anatomical or teardrop implant rotation. Plast Reconstr Surg 109:2555-2564, 2002.
8. Chantal M, Melis P, Marco R. Suturing of a textured breast implant filled with cohesive silicone gel to prevent dislocation. Scand J Plast Reconstr Surg Hand Surg 37:236-238, 2003.

Editorial Commentary

Dr. De Lorenzi has very considerable experience with cohesive gel implants, and when he says that they give the best results in augmentation mammaplasty, then one has to pay careful attention to his words of wisdom. There is absolutely no doubt that, in the case of these implants, the choice of size and shape is paramount. When the procedure is being contemplated, a very comprehensive discussion should be carried out with the patient regarding the implant, how it is inserted, and what is expected of it. In this article the approach to insertion of the implant, the size of the incision, and the position of the implant are spelled out very carefully. Further advice is given on the pocket, particularly about the extent of undermining.

These implants are very different from those used in the past, albeit the very recent past. It is no longer a case of making a pocket and putting the implant into it with virtually no attention being paid to the position of the implant within the pocket. In our experience with previous implants, the size of the pocket was paramount, but the position of the implant, whether saline-filled or silicone-filled, was not a matter of great concern. Retaining the philosophy associated with previously used implants may lead to a virtual disaster if correct technique is not used. With care, gentle technique, and correct placement, a very natural end result can be achieved. With rough technique there can be fracture of the internal gel structure, and, as a result of this, an underlying deformity can occur.

Another factor that has been stressed is that very accurate preoperative assessment should be made, because, when using these implants as Dr. De Lorenzi advocates, the four important factors to be remembered are:

- Choice of implant
- Size of incision
- Size of pocket
- Required shape of the breast

Paying attention to these basic tenets will improve results and help prevent problems.

Ian T. Jackson, MD

Decisions and Applications in Aesthetic and Reconstructive Breast Surgery

João Carlos Sampaio Góes, MD, PhD; Alan Landecker, MD;
Paulo Miranda Godoy, MD; Renata Sampaio Góes, MD

Aesthetic and reconstructive breast surgery can achieve excellent results using modern cohesive silicone gel implants, which have been extensively modified since their introduction in the early 1960s. Plastic surgeons now possess a myriad of options regarding their shape, design, surface, and filler material. These developments have minimized complications, increased safety, and improved the aesthetic results of these operations.

Cohesive silicone gel implants have a natural feel and low potential for capsular contracture, rupture, or rippling. These features have been improved by the latest technical refinements in the approaches, the incisions, and especially the pocket planes. The pocket plane is the most influential factor in the dynamics established between the implant and the soft tissues after surgery. An adequate pocket must be dissected accurately to avoid postoperative displacement of the implant and should have strong enough tissues to support the implant and conceal its borders.

The indications, benefits, and trade-offs of the subglandular, partial retropectoral, and completely submuscular pocket planes have been extensively analyzed in the literature. More recently the development of the subfascial approach (which uses the pectoralis major fascia as an extra unit for implant coverage) has offered more natural long-term outcomes. This conclusion derives from applying this technique in 341 primary and secondary patients since 1994 and the extensive experience of the senior author (JCSG) with ablation of breast cancer and breast reconstruction.

In this chapter we present the most important aspects of surgical technique, benefits, trade-offs, and outcomes of the subfascial approach in primary and secondary breast augmentation and in immediate breast reconstruction using silicone cohesive gel implants.

ANATOMY

The pectoral fascia, a thin layer of tissue that lies over the pectoralis major muscle, is attached to the sternum and the clavicle; it is continuous with the fascia of the shoulder, axilla, and thorax inferolaterally. At the caudal border of the pectoralis major muscle the clavipectoral, pectoral, and serratus anterior fasciae become continuous and form suspensory ligaments that extend to the breast's inframammary fold and its investing fascia. The pectoralis fascia may be used as an additional coverage and stabilizing system for the upper pole of breast implants, offering more natural long-term outcomes.

SUBFASCIAL APPROACH IN PRIMARY AND SECONDARY BREAST AUGMENTATION

Breast augmentation has enjoyed worldwide acceptance in the last few decades because of continued improvements of modern implants, refinement of surgical techniques, and cultural trends that emphasize exposure of the body. To optimize the outcomes of this operation, factors such as incision location, pocket plane, implant design, and individual tissue characteristics must be carefully considered. Satisfactory results depend on adjusting available options to each patient's requirements.

Advantages and Disadvantages of Subfascial Augmentation

The subfascial breast augmentation technique using cohesive silicone gel implants offers excellent long-term aesthetic results because the dynamics between the implant and soft tissues have been optimized. Additionally, important aspects of this operation, such as morbidity and postoperative recovery, have been minimized. This technique is extremely versatile and may be used for primary breast augmentation and for patients requiring removal or replacement of implants.

The creation of a strong support system for the implant's superior pole is the technique's main feature. Displacement of the implant in the superior direction is avoided because its upper pole is placed between the muscle and the fascia, which constitutes a stronger supporting system than just the breast parenchyma and/or subcutaneous tissue in the conventional submammary approach. The subfascial technique also helps the implant's upper half retain its shape and position over time and helps conceal its borders. A natural outcome is generated because the skin and subcutaneous tissue in the upper half of the pocket are not directly in contact with the implant, allowing the skin and subcutaneous layers to move freely and independently as a separate system.

The subfascial technique enables the surgeon to combine the potential benefits of the subglandular approach (such as accurate control of both breast shape and inframammary fold position, rapid postoperative recovery, and lack of distortion during pectoralis muscle contraction) with an increased amount of tissue available to cover the implant's upper pole. Although the fascia offers less tissue for coverage than the pectoralis major muscle, we feel that some of the potential benefits of using the pectoralis major have been achieved. Also, trade-offs of the subpectoral approach, such as a tendency for lateral and superior displacement of implants over time, visible changes of breast shape during contraction of the muscle, increased morbidity in terms of pain and recovery, and less control over the inframammary fold's position, have been significantly reduced when compared with the subglandular approach.

Dissection of the entire pocket in the subfascial plane has several disadvantages. First, concealing the implant borders in the lower third of the breast may not be significantly enhanced in patients with a thin and fragile fascia in this area. Second, morbidity may be enhanced by factors such as extended operating time and increased potential for bleeding, because dissection of the pocket in the subfascial plane is slower than in the conventional submammary plane and requires more meticulous hemostasis. The use of a high-frequency electrocautery with a needle tip or an ultrasonic scalpel obviates this potential problem. In our experience, the benefits of the subfascial approach have been much more significant than these potential trade-offs.

PLANNING
Pocket Plane Selection

In breast augmentation, pocket plane selection is perhaps the most influential factor in the dynamics established between an implant and soft tissues after surgery. Before the development of the subfascial approach the most commonly employed pocket planes were subglandular, partial retropectoral, and totally submuscular. The indications, benefits, and trade-offs of these strategies have been extensively analyzed in the literature.

After performing numerous cohesive gel implant operations using the conventional submammary approach, we observed that the implant's superior border had a tendency to project in the anterior direction after variable time periods. This caused somewhat unnatural results in previously pleasing outcomes because the implant's border could be seen. Clearly a more stable coverage system was required to avoid this problem.

Use of the subfascial plane has become increasingly popular since it was reported by authors performing transaxillary breast augmentation. In general, the pectoralis major fascia tends to be thin and more fragile over the lower half of the pectoralis major muscle. The progressive thickening of the fascia along the upper half of the muscle constitutes the basis of the subfascial augmentation technique. The strong supporting system offered by the thickened fascia in the superior and medial regions of the breast gives excellent coverage and concealment of the implant borders in these areas, offering natural long-term outcomes. Therefore, in the subfascial approach, the anterior wall of the implant's pocket consists of the pectoral fascia, breast parenchyma, subcutaneous tissue, and skin.

Incisions and Approaches

The operation is performed under general anesthesia without infiltration. The choice of approach and incision (or incisions) should be based on a thorough discussion with the patient regarding her preference and the advantages and trade-offs of each option. For patients desiring a periareolar approach, the incision location depends on whether a change in the position of the areola is anticipated and on the diameter of the areola. We find that the periareolar approach generally results in scars that are excellent and become inconspicuous after the maturation process. Another advantage is that it establishes a central easy access to all regions of the breast, which may be especially helpful in patients having secondary procedures that require capsulotomy or capsulectomy.

For patients whose areola is in a satisfactory position, the incision should be placed in the lower half of the areola. In patients requiring extensive elevation of the areola or breast tissues, the incision should be placed along the upper half of the areola and may be combined with a circumferential periareolar, vertical, or inverted T incision if necessary. Other approaches should be used when the diameter of the patient's areola is too small for the implant.

The inframammary approach offers advantages such as easy access, nondisruption of the breast's parenchyma, and allowing the use of virtually any type or size of implant. It also facilitates accurate dissection and hemostasis of the pocket. The incision is usually 4 cm long and should be located slightly lateral to the inferior projection of the nipple-areolar complex on the inframammary fold and approximately 0.5 cm above the anticipated new fold.

In the senior author's experience, the axillary and transumbilical approaches may not be appropriate when using cohesive silicone gel implants. The axillary approach may result in an unaesthetic scar that may be problematic in countries where exposure of the body is frequent. Also, hemostasis is a challenge, it is difficult to create an accurate pocket, and there may be an increased tendency for superior displacement of the implant with time because of inaccurate release of the pectoralis major muscle at the inframammary fold area. Other disadvantages are that endoscopic instruments are frequently required, and it may be difficult to insert the bulky cohesive silicone gel implants through a relatively small and distant access site.

The transumbilical approach possesses most of the same disadvantages of the axillary approach, and insertion of cohesive gel implants through the umbilicus is virtually impossible.

TECHNIQUE
Dissection of the Subfascial Pocket

When the incision is in the lower hemisphere of the areola, dissection should be performed in the caudal direction parallel to the skin (as in skin-sparing mastectomies) for approximately 4 cm. After dissection, the breast's parenchyma is incised in a radial direction (perpendicular to the skin incision) and vertically until the muscle layer is reached (Fig. 1). This avoids any communication between the skin and the parenchymal incisions. After inserting the implant, closing the incised tissues establishes a relatively secure isolation of the implant from the atmosphere, reducing the risk of infection.

Additionally, radial dissection of the breast's parenchyma facilitates the adjustment of glandular flaps for breast shaping in patients undergoing tumor resection or when ptosis and insufficient upper-pole fullness are present.

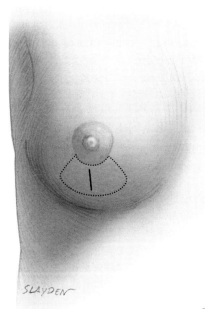
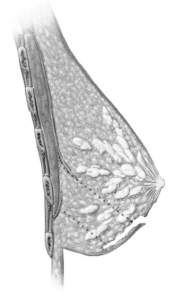

FIG. 1

After the pectoralis major muscle layer is reached, dissection of the implant pocket is performed in the subfascial plane using either high-frequency electrocautery with a needle tip or an ultrasonic scalpel. The anterior wall of the implant pocket using the subfascial approach should consist of pectoral fascia, breast parenchyma, subcutaneous tissue, and skin. The fascia is sufficiently thick in the superior and medial poles of the breast to offer an additional anatomic structure to cover the implant (Fig. 2).

It is very important to create a pocket with adequate dimensions that allow the implant to lie comfortably inside. An accurately sized pocket results in improved adherence between soft tissues and the implant's surface. A pocket that is too small may lead to compression of the implant, creation of folds, and unaesthetic distortions of the breast's shape. Excessively large pockets may cause displacement of the implant and accumulation of liquid.

If necessary, the inframammary fold should be lowered so that the horizontal middle axis of the implant is centered on the nipple. The amount of lowering correlates with the implant's diameter. When doing this, the attachments of the fascia to the skin at the level of the fold must be disrupted to avoid deformities such as high-riding implants and double-bubble contours in the lower breast. Undermining should not extend laterally beyond the lateral breast border to avoid injury to the fourth and fifth intercostal nerves that innervate the nipple-areolar complex. This also avoids lateral displacement of the implant after surgery.

After meticulous hemostasis has been achieved, the implants are bathed in cephalothin (Keflin) solution and inserted into the pockets. The preferred implants are anatomic cohesive gel implants with a textured surface. Layered wound closure is performed using Vicryl and Monocryl subdermal sutures and Monocryl intradermal sutures. Suction drains are inserted, usually through the axilla, and are removed when the output is less than 30 ml per day on each side. The suction system also helps maximize adherence between the pocket's soft tissues and the implant's surface.

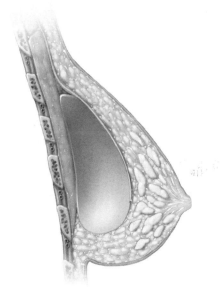

FIG. 2

At the end of the operation it is important to assess the positions of the implants in relation to each other and to the thoracic wall. In general, the distance between the areola's inferior border and the inframammary fold should be approximately 6 to 7 cm (called x). The distance between the areola's superior border and the uppermost point of the breast should be approximately 9 to 10.5 cm (or $1.5x$). Two other important parameters are the distances between the implants and between each areola's medial border and the midsternal line. Appropriate distances are 2 to 3 cm and 9 to 10 cm, respectively.

Dressing and Postoperative Care

At the end of the operation, adhesive dressings are placed around the breast in a triangular fashion (similar to a bra) to shape, support, and compress the soft tissues somewhat. These are removed after about 5 days. An elastic band or strap should be used over the superior poles of the breasts for 2 weeks to avoid superior displacement of the implants, keep the newly created inframammary fold in the desired position, and expand the tissues in the inferior pole of the breast. Massaging or moving the breasts should be avoided for at least 4 weeks to avoid detaching the soft tissues of the pocket from the surface of the implant, which may lead to an accumulation of liquid.

Special Clinical Situations
Secondary Breast Augmentation

During secondary breast augmentation, or for patients requiring removal of submuscular implants, new implants should be placed in the subfascial plane whenever possible. Capsulectomy and fixation of the pectoralis muscle to the thorax are routinely performed in these cases to avoid creating a pocket and accumulating liquid, which may be a source of infection and/or other complications.

Segmental Pectoralis Major Muscle Flap

For very thin patients, for those requesting larger implants, and for patients who present with rippling, harvesting part of the pectoralis major muscle may be necessary to help conceal the implant's borders in the superomedial pole of the breast because the coverage offered by the subfascial approach alone may not be sufficient.

In these patients a segmental pectoralis major muscle flap, based on perforators located along the sternal border, is raised, placed along and over the implant's superomedial pole, and sutured to the underlying pectoralis muscle (Fig. 3). The flap is generally 15 cm long and 4 cm wide. With this approach lateral or superior dislocation of the implant resulting from contraction of the pectoralis muscle (frequently seen with submuscular augmentation) is avoided because only a strip of the muscle is used.

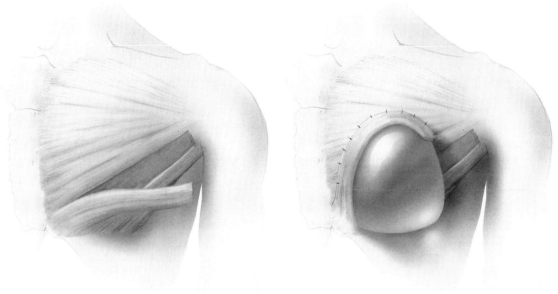

FIG. 3

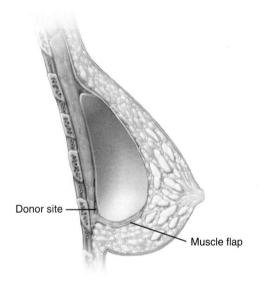

FIG. 4

Inferior Myofascial Flap

The pectoralis major muscle fascia may be used to treat patients who have excessive caudal migration of breast implants. After removing the implants, the fascia and/or muscle 2 to 4 cm above the planned inframammary fold is dissected, creating a small inferiorly based flap (Fig. 4). Placing the implant under this flap strengthens the supporting system of the inferior part of the implant and may help secure the implant in place after fixation of the inframammary fold in its correct position.

RESULTS

Pleasing results have been obtained using the techniques described here, including a natural breast shape, a smooth transition between soft tissue and implant in the supero-medial pole, and low morbidity. The rate of capsular contracture has been extremely low, and there have been no complaints regarding displacement of the implants during contraction of the pectoralis major muscle.

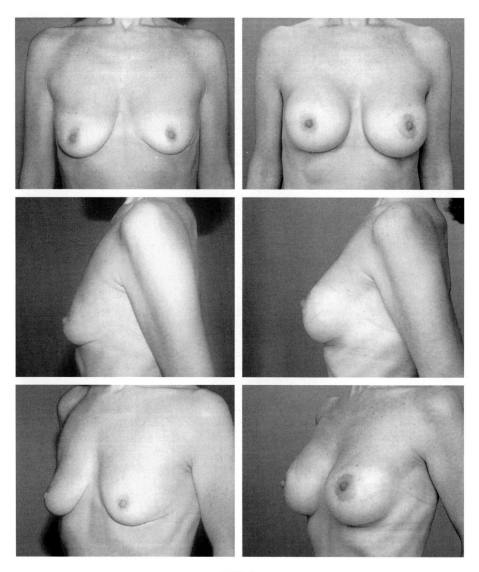

FIG. 5

This 36-year-old patient had breast augmentation with 280 cc anatomic implants in the subfascial plane using a periareolar approach. Her results are shown after 1 year. Augmentation produced satisfactory elevation of the areolas and filling of the skin envelope, achieving natural results.

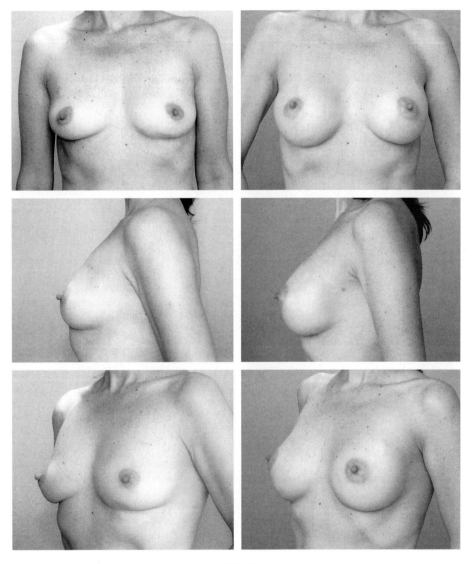

FIG. 6

This 31-year-old patient had breast augmentation with 270 cc anatomic implants in the subfascial plane using an inframammary approach. Her results are shown after 1 year. The subfascial approach allowed concealment of the implant's superomedial border bilaterally.

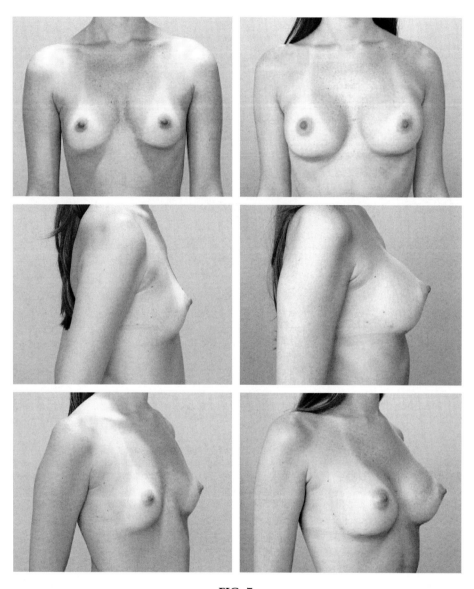

FIG. 7

This 29-year-old patient had breast augmentation with 320 cc anatomic implants in the subfascial plane using an inframammary approach. Results are shown after 1 year. With thin patients relatively larger implants can achieve excellent results using the subfascial approach.

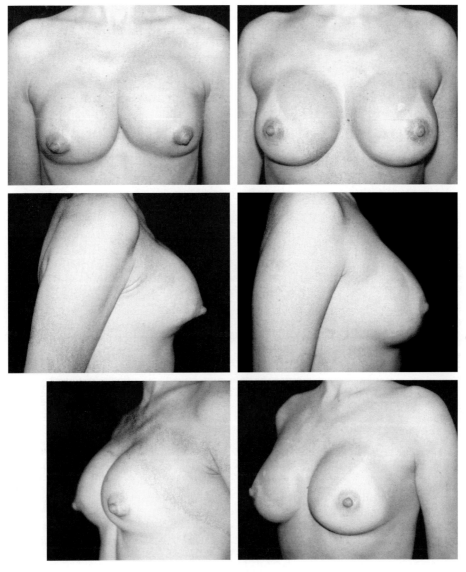

FIG. 8

This patient presented with significant capsular contracture. Her implants were re-moved and new 270 cc anatomic implants were placed in the subfascial plane. A seg-mental pectoralis major flap was used to protect the implant's upper pole. Results are shown after 6 months. Improved symmetry of the inframammary folds and areolas was obtained, as well as correction of the symmastia.

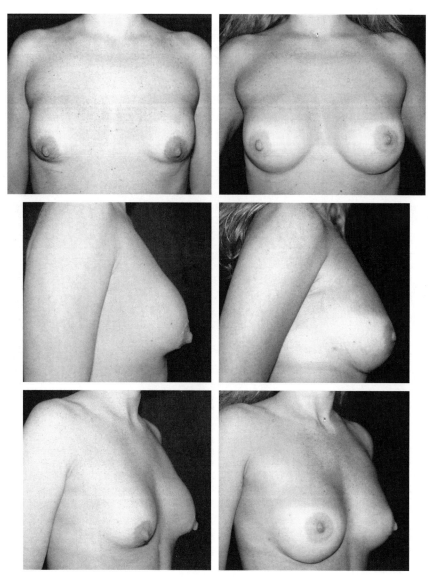

FIG. 9

This patient presented with displacement of submuscular breast implants. The original implants were removed and new 270 cc anatomic implants were placed in the subfascial plane. Results are shown after 6 months. The inframammary fold was lowered into the correct position, which corrected the Snoopy deformity by elevating the areolas.

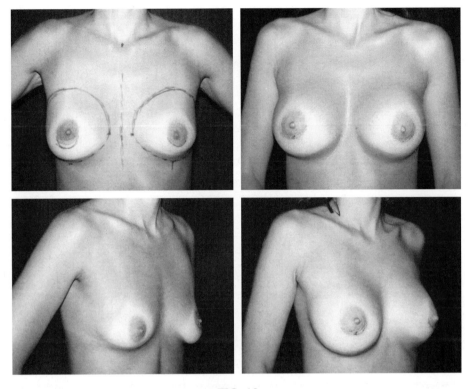

FIG. 10

This 36-year-old patient had breast augmentation with 270 cc anatomic implants in the subfascial plane using an inframammary approach. Results are shown after 1 year. Satisfactory augmentation was obtained by concealing the implants' borders in the superomedial regions of the breasts.

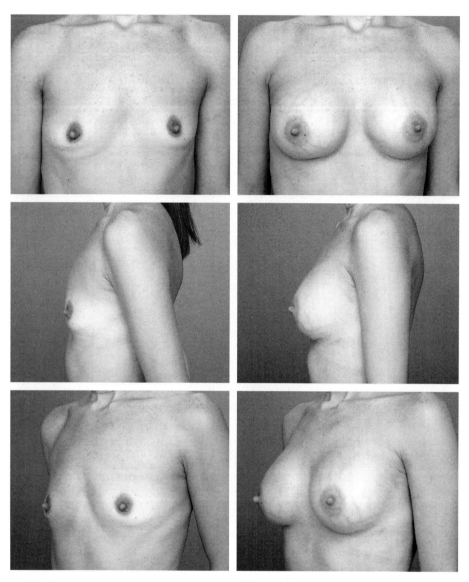

FIG. 11

This 42-year-old patient had breast augmentation with 280 cc anatomic implants in the subfascial plane using an inframammary approach. Results are shown after 1 year. The implants filled the redundant skin envelope with natural results.

BREAST RECONSTRUCTION WITH COHESIVE GEL IMPLANTS

In breast reconstruction with cohesive gel implants the greatest challenge is to offer patients satisfactory long-term aesthetic results. These results depend greatly on the type, quality, and amount of tissue available to cover the implant. Unfortunately, long-term outcomes such as visible implant borders, capsular contracture, and unnatural shape are relatively common. This occurs because the amount of local tissue available to cover an implant is reduced by removing glandular tissue and the pectoralis major fascia during the mastectomy procedure. Additionally, local tissues have a remarkable tendency to thin out over time, decreasing the quality of coverage.

These problems have led us to recognize a need to harvest additional tissue to improve coverage. Most traditional techniques include using autologous flaps for coverage, but these flaps create additional (and often significant) donor site morbidity. Although results often look natural, the consistency of the new tissue is not always similar to breast tissue.

To address these problems, the senior author began using laparoscopically harvested omental flaps for breast reconstruction in 1995. In this technique, the omentum on the right gastroepiploic pedicle is mobilized laparoscopically through a 4 cm midline incision in the aponeurosis of the superior epigastric region. The aponeurosis is also opened laparoscopically, obviating the need for an external epigastric incision and further reducing donor site morbidity. The omental flap is tunneled subcutaneously toward the mastectomy site where it can be used to restore the breast's volume.

Since this technique was first used, it has been adapted and refined to help cover cohesive gel implants in most patients undergoing this type of reconstruction. The omental flap serves as a substitute for the removed breast parenchyma. It can be used exclusively or with synthetic mesh when a partial submuscular technique is used.

Operative Procedures
Exclusive Omental Flap Coverage

The exclusive omental flap coverage technique is used most frequently in previously augmented patients who have developed breast cancer. These patients require autologous tissue to replace the breast parenchyma after it is excised through a periareolar mastectomy. During the ablative procedure, the implant's capsule should be left intact whenever possible (unless removal is indicated for oncologic reasons), because it helps support and maintain the implant in position. This is important because the omentum alone does not offer enough tissue to completely cover and support an anatomic cohesive gel implant.

Restoration of the breast's volume is accomplished by covering the original implant and capsule using the pedicled omentum and the native breast skin. This is performed by folding the omentum over itself until it resembles the breast cone and fixing it to the inframammary fold and underlying muscle with 3-0 Monocryl sutures. It is important to ensure that the entire implant is adequately and securely covered by the omentum, which has replaced the breast parenchyma (Figs. 12 and 13).

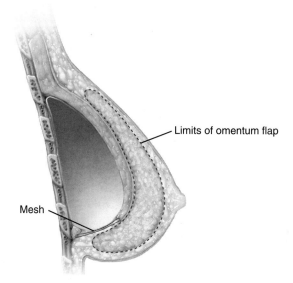

FIG. 12

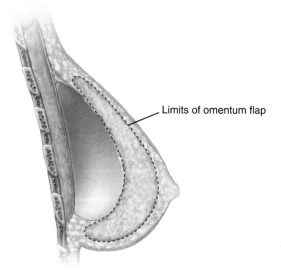

FIG. 13

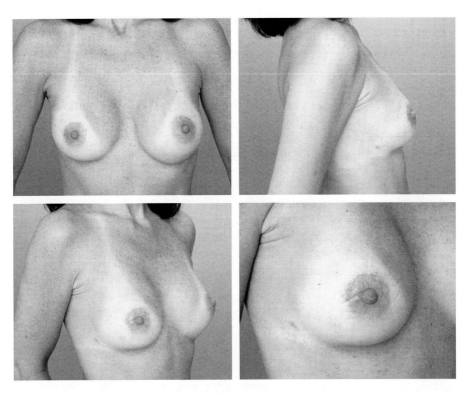

FIG. 14

This 34-year-old patient underwent an exclusive omental flap reconstruction technique on the right breast. She is shown postoperatively.

Partial Submuscular Technique With Synthetic Mesh and Omental Flap Coverage

The partial submuscular technique using synthetic mesh and omental flap coverage may be used in patients whose primary breast reconstruction is to be performed using anatomic cohesive gel implants. It may also be used in patients who have small omental flaps or who require bilateral reconstruction, because the omentum alone may not offer sufficient tissue for adequate and secure coverage of the anatomic cohesive gel implants. This technique may also be used with previously augmented patients who require removal and replacement of implants and their capsules for oncologic reasons.

In this technique the upper two thirds of the implants should be placed in the submuscular plane. A customized piece of synthetic Vipro II mesh is sutured to the inferior border of the muscle and then to the inframammary fold using 4-0 nylon sutures so that the lower third of the implant is entirely covered and supported (see Fig. 13). Using mesh in the stabilizing system helps maintain the implant in position and avoids some of the problems commonly seen in patients who have undergone submuscular breast augmentation: retraction of the pectoralis muscle in the superior direction during contraction, lateral and superior displacement of the implants over time, and visible changes of breast shape during contraction of the muscle. The coverage system is completed using the omentum, which is divided so that approximately half of the flap covers each implant in bilateral reconstruction cases, and native breast skin, as described previously.

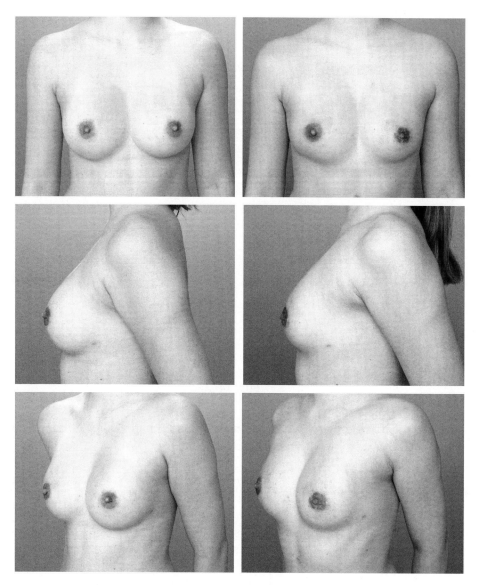

FIG. 15

Here may be seen preoperative and 1-year postoperative views of a 34-year-old patient who underwent bilateral breast reconstruction using the partial submuscular technique with synthetic mesh and omental flap coverage.

The technique for breast reconstruction using anatomic cohesive gel implants and the omental flap has significant advantages. First, the omentum is a pedicled flap with an abundant and safe blood supply. The pedicle's length (approximately 12 cm) ensures that the flap reaches the mastectomy site without tension. Second, the omentum provides efficient coverage for the implant and has a consistency similar to the breast parenchyma. These factors are responsible for extremely reliable and natural long-term outcomes. Third, donor site morbidity is significantly reduced by harvesting the flap laparoscopically, which leaves the patient only with the scars related to the laparoscopy procedure. In the recipient site, only a periareolar scar remains in most patients because periareolar mastectomy (which preserves the native breast skin) is the preferred ablative approach. These factors ensure a less-aggressive operation with a shorter hospital stay and a more comfortable postoperative recovery. The few disadvantages include the learning curve, need for laparoscopic equipment, and the risks related to intraabdominal operations.

SUGGESTED READINGS

Abbes MJL, Richelme H, Demard F. The greater omentum in repair of complications following surgery and radiotherapy for certain cancers. Int Surg 59:81, 1974.

Argenta LC. Reconstruction of the breast by tissue expansion. Clin Plast Surg 11:257, 1984.

Arnold PG, Hartrampf CR, Jurkiewicz MJ. One-stage reconstruction of the breast using the transposed greater omentum: Case report. Plast Reconstr Surg 57:520, 1976.

Barnett A. Transaxillary subpectoral augmentation in the ptotic breast: Augmentation by disruption of the extended pectoral fascia and parenchymal sweep. Plast Reconstr Surg 86:76, 1990.

Biggs TM, Yarish RS. Augmentation mammaplasty: Retropectoral versus retromammary implantation. Clin Plast Surg 15:549, 1988.

Bostwick J III, Nahai F, Wallace JG, et al. Sixty latissimus dorsi flaps. Plast Reconstr Surg 63:31, 1979.

Bostwick J, Vasconez LO, Jurkiewicz MJ. Breast reconstruction after a radical mastectomy. Plast Reconstr Surg 61:682, 1978.

Cort DF, Collis JL. Omental transposition in the treatment of radionecrosis. Br J Surg 60:580, 1973.

Dempsey WC, Latham WD. Subpectoral implants in augmentation mammaplasty: Preliminary report. Plast Reconstr Surg 42:515, 1968.

Dowden RV, Horton CE, Rosato FE, et al. Reconstruction of the breast after mastectomy for cancer. Surg Gynecol Obstet 149:109, 1979.

Dupont C, Menard Y. Transposition of the greater omentum for reconstruction of the chest wall. Plast Reconstr Surg 49:263, 1972.

Elliott LF, Beegle PH, Hartrampf CR. The lateral transverse thigh free flap: An alternative for autogenous-tissue breast reconstruction. Plast Reconstr Surg 85:169, 1990.

Elliott LF, Hartramph CR. Breast reconstruction: Progress in the past decade. World J Surg 14:763, 1990.

Erol OO, Spira M. Reconstructing the breast mound employing a secondary island omental skin flap. Plast Reconstr Surg 86:510, 1990.

Góes JCS. Breast reconstruction following mastectomy: Who, when and how. Breast Diseases 5:4, 1979.

Góes JCS. Periareolar mammaplasty: Double skin technique. Breast Dis 4:111, 1991.

Góes JCS, Landecker A. Optimizing outcomes in breast augmentation: Seven years of experience with the subfascial plane. Aesthetic Plast Surg 27:178, 2003.

Graf RM, Bernardes A, Auersvald A, et al. Subfascial endoscopic transaxillary augmentation mammaplasty. Aesthetic Plast Surg 24:216, 2000.

Gray H. Gray's Anatomy, 37th ed. London: Churchill Livingstone, 1989.

Hidalgo DA. Breast Augmentation: Choosing the optimal incision, implant, and pocket plane. Plast Reconstr Surg 105:2202, 2000.

Mahler D, Ben-Yakar J, Hauben DJ. The retropectoral route for breast augmentation. Aesthetic Plast Surg 6:237, 1982.

Papillon J. Pros and cons of subpectoral implantation. Clin Plast Surg 3:321, 1976.

Puckett CL, Croll GH, Reichel CA, et al. A critical look at capsular contracture in subglandular versus subpectoral mammary augmentation. Aesthetic Plast Surg 11:23, 1987.

Regnault P. Partially submuscular breast augmentation. Plast Reconstr Surg 59:72, 1977.

Tebbetts JB. Dual plane breast augmentation: Optimizing implant-soft-tissue relationships in a wide range of breast types. Plast Reconstr Surg 107:1255, 2001.

Tebbetts JB. Transaxillary subpectoral augmentation mammaplasty: Long-term follow-up and refinements. Plast Reconstr Surg 74:636, 1984.

Editorial Commentary

Dr. Góes and his colleagues feel that placing an implant in the subfascial plane, having dissected a pocket above the pectoralis, optimizes the dynamics between the implant and the soft tissues. They feel that the morbidity and the postoperative recovery period are decreased, and that there is a very strong support system between the muscle and overlying fascia. One of the points they emphasize is that a more subtle superior pole can result. They also feel that the borders of the implant are rather more concealed.

It is interesting that here is a group that has come from preferring the submuscular position to preferring a supermuscle subfascial position. This is where the cohesive gel implant of the right shape can give a very acceptable result, as opposed to previous saline-filled or silicone-filled implants. Being able to place an implant in a more superficial position and end up with excellent results, as these authors show, illustrates the dependability of shape and position of these implants when used as directed.

There are times, as we would all agree, that the cover for our implant varies according to the patient's breast and what we want to achieve. The information provided by this group of authors helps greatly in terms of this decision-making. It is reassuring to know that the implants may be covered with omentum or synthetic mesh, or in this case Vicryl mesh. I believe in the latter situation we might well want to consider the use of Alloderm (LifeCell Corp, Branchburg, NJ). The authors have used a periareolar approach when indicated, but they point out, as we know, that this cannot always be used. The situation when they have attempted to use an axillary approach is similar.

In this article, using cohesive gel implants in reconstruction for postmastectomy patients is considered. I have no doubt that this technique is successful.

Ian T. Jackson, MD

Dr. Góes and colleagues discuss the relationship between implant position and outcome, making a convincing argument that subfascial augmentation has benefits despite having a slower dissection with more potential bleeding. The overall benefits include better support for the upper pole as well as better overall shape and breast dynamics during patient movement. I use the subfascial approach regularly for primary augmentations in selected patients. It is my experience that the main advantage of the subfascial approach is that the edge of the device in the upper pole is well hidden. This is because the fascia is tightly held to the pectoralis muscle by vertical fibers that intermingle with the muscle fibers. These fibers contain many small blood vessels, making this dissection quite tedious and prone to more bleeding than the relatively quick and avascular subpectoral dissection. However, the surgeon is rewarded because the nonextensile fascial layer applies some mild compression at the edge of the upper pole and prevents soft tissue retraction. This provides control for the edge of the device so that the skin does not curve under the edge of the implant, thus preventing the "Baywatch breast." The subfascial approach should not be used if there is insufficient tissue coverage for submammary augmentation. If sufficient tissue is not present, then a submuscular approach is mandatory, because a subfascial approach will not prevent deformities. A range of tissue thickness is usually suggested, because part of the decision for using submuscular versus submammary placement involves measurements that are accurate only to within several millimeters. There is also a difference in the quality of tissues—whether thin and stretched with striae distensae or thick and never having been stretched—so that there is always room for sound clinical judgement. Also a word of caution that these techniques were developed with appropriately sized devices matched to patient measurements. If oversized devices are used, it is likely that the deformities will occur. Dr. Góes' group describes pectoralis flaps that may be useful to a surgeon dealing with thin atrophic tissues, such as with the unfortunate sequelae from overprojecting implants. These flaps are also useful for aesthetic surgery patients who have complications requiring soft tissue coverage either at the implant border or inferiorly, when a vascularized muscle flap can bring tissue where it is needed to achieve a good result. These authors also describe their experience using omentum to replace breast parenchyma removed to treat malignancy. Finally, they discuss the use of alloplastic mesh material for support, which may be used in combination with the other techniques. I have no personal experience with these methods.

Claudio De Lorenzi, BA, MD

Breast Augmentation Using an Inframammary Incision

Rolf R. Olbrisch, MD

Augmentation mammaplasty with cohesive gel implants provides a stable and precise method for breast reshaping. Although several surgical approaches are available for implant insertion, the inframammary approach has decided benefits. This incision allows access for manipulating the fascia and musculature and affords an excellent view of the implant pocket to achieve hemostasis and ensure proper implant positioning before closure. An inframammary fold incision also permits the use of implants of all sizes and shapes.

INCISION PLACEMENT

The distance from the new inframammary fold position to the border of the areola has to be measured and taken into consideration when the inframammary incision is chosen. Because the fold will move downward when the breast volume increases, the incision line must be located at the future position of the fold so that the scar will be hidden.

RETROGLANDULAR OR RETROPECTORAL IMPLANTATION

Both retroglandular and retropectoral placement of an implant can be easily achieved through an inframammary incision line. Patients desire a well-hidden implant; therefore the surgeon must decide whether, with retroglandular positioning, there will be sufficient overlying tissue to hide the implant. If a pinch test reveals 2 cm of tissue thickness, the implant may be placed retroglandularly to create a natural-seeming breast, because tissue is replaced where it is lacking.

Retropectoral placement leads to a volume gain under the pectoralis muscle, which is less natural but nevertheless mandatory if the patient is very thin and the implant cannot be hidden under breast tissue. Although creating a retroglandular pocket is fairly painless and associated with reduced bleeding, the retropectoral implantation needs greater surgical intervention in the anatomic structures, because the pectoralis muscle must be released from its origin on the sternum. Dissection of the muscle may lead to a higher incidence of bleeding and greater postoperative pain.

The historical advice to massage the implant is no longer valid, because cohesive gel implants may have a textured surface that may allow ingrowth of tissue. Massage would be counterproductive to this process. The complication of implants moving caudally to create a double-bubble phenomenon occurs only in retropectoral implants. If the pectoralis major muscle is not adequately released from its origin on the sternum, the breast can show deformities when the muscle is activated, especially in athletic women.

PATIENT EVALUATION
Anatomic Considerations

Breast aesthetics is dependent on the size and shape of the breasts, as well as their relationship to the body, thorax, and hips. When performing augmentation mammaplasty it is essential to keep these relationships in mind. They will influence the size, shape, and placement of the implants. For example, thoracic deformities can make it necessary to choose different implant sizes for each breast. To help determine the proper placement choice for an implant, whether retroglandular or subpectoral, the breast tissue is examined above the areola with a pinch test. A thickness of two fingers allows placement over the muscle.

In some patients the surgeon will find challenges such as the following:
- Anorexic patients with an extremely thin layer of tissue covering the implant that will likely exhibit implant edges
- Androgynous patients or intense body-builders with hypertrophic pectoralis muscles and no underlying fatty tissue
- Asymmetry because of rippling
- Patients who want bigger implants
- Patients with deformities caused by capsular contracture
- Patients in whom an implant had to be temporarily removed because of infection

PLANNING
Measurements

The following measurements must be taken (with the skin stretched):
- The jugulum-areola distance (assuming a typical areola diameter of 4.5 cm)
- The width of the breast
- The areola–inframammary fold distance, which generally requires a mastopexy if the distance is more than 7 cm

The distances measured and the volume and shape of the original breast dictate the shape and size of implant chosen. For example, a breast width of 10 cm will need an implant 10 cm wide. A wider implant will result in deformity.

Markings

Preoperative planning and marking are performed with the patient in a standing position or in a sitting position on the OR table (Fig. 1).

First the midline of the thorax is marked. The inframammary folds and the contours of each entire breast are marked using the other hand to gently shift the breast tissue to the skin borders (Fig. 2).

The distances between the jugulum and the areola and between the areola and the inframammary fold are compared on each side (Fig. 3). A bra cup size of B requires a distance of 5 cm from the areola to the inframammary fold, C needs 5.5 to 6 cm, and D needs up to 7 cm and a possible periareolar mastopexy after augmentation. This means that the inframammary fold will shift downward when the breast volume increases.

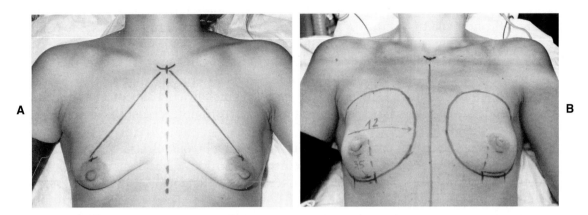

FIG. 1   **A,** The jugulum-areola distance is marked to determine possible ptosis. Here the distance is 19 cm, which is within the normal range. The middle of the thorax is also marked. **B,** Begin marking with the patient asleep in the sitting position. The contour of the breast is marked to determine the implant borders.

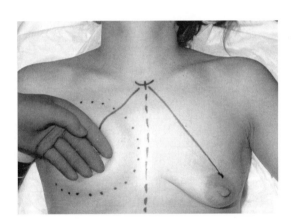

FIG. 2   The breast is shifted to the sides to determine the borders of the breast. This is especially useful with very small breasts. Note the markings indicating the borders.

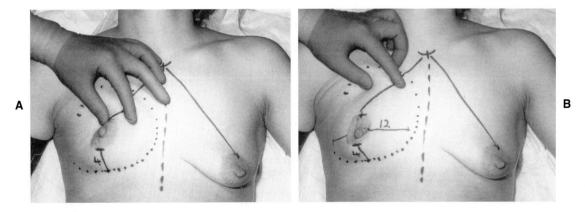

FIG. 3   **A,** The distance between the inframammary fold and the areola complex is shown, which is 4 cm in this patient. **B,** The breast width in this patient is 12 cm. This measurement is important in helping choose the right implant width. The implant width should be no more than 0.5 cm less than the breast width.

The incision line is marked in the newly planned inframammary fold. It must be determined exactly so that it will be hidden in the new fold. The incision begins at the point on the new fold that vertically aligns with the medial areola rim and is 4.5 to 5 cm in length, depending on the size of the implant (Fig. 4).

The perforators should be marked so that the surgeon can better anticipate their locations when operating, because if they bleed they must be coagulated (Fig. 5).

The patient is positioned supine on the operating table with a supporting knee roll and cushioned heels. Her arms should be at her side to promote a smooth dissection to a relaxed pectoralis muscle.

Instruments such as an extended Bovie tip and a long bipolar electric forceps for coagulation will ensure a smooth operative course. In addition, a headlight or lighted retractor will make all parts of the implant pocket accessible and visible so that necessary bleeding control is achieved effectively.

Injecting anesthesia with adrenaline in the incision line helps minimize bleeding during creation of the pocket. Sometimes it is useful to inject approximately 100 cc of tumescent solution to facilitate creation of the pocket.

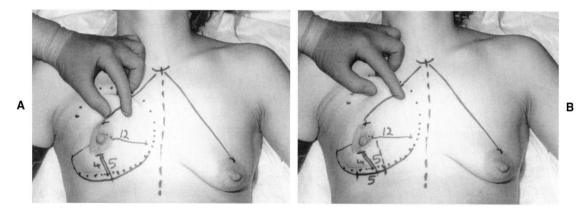

FIG. 4   A, The new inframammary fold is marked at 5 cm. **B,** A 5 cm inframammary incision is marked.

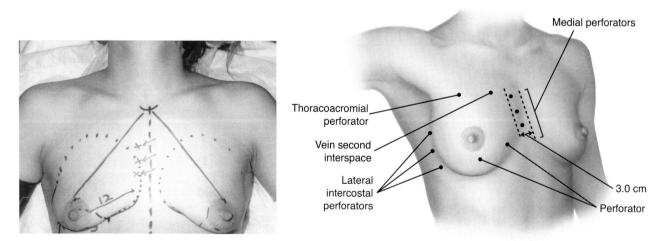

FIG. 5   The most important and consistent perforators are marked.

SURGICAL TECHNIQUE

The skin incision is made with a No. 15 blade. Sharp dissection of the subcutaneous tissue continues with the 15 blade or a cautery blade until the fascia of the thorax is encountered and the border of the breast tissue and muscle is revealed. When the edge of the muscle is clearly identified, the pocket is developed either retroglandularly or subpectorally. Blunt dissection with the index finger helps reduce bleeding because the vessels contract by intimal spasm. Fibrotic fibers are dissected sharply with the cautery blade and with the help of a headlight. The pocket is created so that it precisely follows the preoperative markings of the borders of the breast. To check the created pocket, the surgeon's index and middle fingers can be used to seal the incision and hold air in the pocket. The ballooned pocket will exhibit every irregularity and provide the surgeon with guidance for more precise dissection.

Care should be taken not to dissect too much on the lateral border of the breast (Fig. 6). The cranial border should be 1 to 2 cm longer than the implant to avoid kinking the implant, which creates a deformed breast with a visible edge. The size of the pocket should be slightly larger than the implant to avoid wrinkles but not large enough to cause rotation and shifting of the implant. A sizer implant is useful if the patient has two different breast shapes or volumes or if the size is not easily determined during preoperative planning.

Bleeding is controlled with bipolar forceps; moist towels are placed in the pocket and the other pocket is created. When the towels are removed they will reveal any residual bleeders.

A 10- to 12-gauge drain is recommended and is mandatory for a secondary implant exchange. It is placed laterocranially in the axilla in the caudal border of the pocket extending into the region of the sternum. The wound is irrigated with a minimum of 200 ml Ringer's lactate solution, and there should be no residual bleeding.

If a subpectoral pocket is necessary, the rim of the muscle should be identified and digitally dissected to the border of the sternum. Here the muscle has to be dissected sharply from the medial border until the height of the areola is reached. The complete dissection can be checked again digitally and should show subcutaneous fat. The borders of the implant pocket can be dissected accordingly.

If the implant is to be completely covered with muscle, the dissection needs to begin in the region of the lateral border of the serratus anterior muscle above the sixth rib. The incision is made there and the muscle is dissected. The cranial border of the muscle is elevated with forceps, and the muscle is elevated using scissors. At the beginning of the fifth rib a digital dissection can be performed to create the pocket.

Implantation is performed with the "no-touch" technique. During this procedure the surgeon changes gloves, and the scrub nurse passes the implant in its inner package

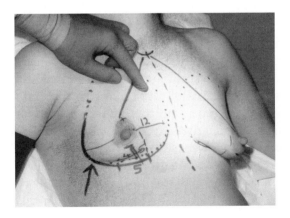

FIG. 6   It is especially important to maintain the lateral border, otherwise the implant can be displaced laterally toward the latissimus border.

without touching it. Povidone-iodine solution is poured over the implant and the incision lines are again cleaned with povidone-iodine solution. The retractor is also bathed in povidone-iodine solution before holding the wound open. The implant is inserted into a sterile plastic bag to avoid skin contact and pushed into the pocket while constantly controlling its position. The drain, not yet connected, eases the insertion by letting air out of the pocket. The exact position of the anatomic implant can be determined by the marking point on the implant. The surgeon's index finger is used to straighten the implant, correcting any folds and checking that the implant pocket is the right size. If the pocket is too small, then a retractor must be used to move the implant aside while the pocket is cut larger. If the pocket is too large, then the implant must be removed, and the pocket must be made smaller using nonresorbable stitches.

After the second implant is inserted, the patient is placed in an upright position and the surgeon checks breast symmetry from the side and front. In most cases further correction can be performed bluntly with a finger while protecting the implant with a spatula.

Each pocket is closed in three layers. A 3-0 Monocryl suture is used to close the thoracic fascia and the fascia of the breast tissue at the height of the new inframammary fold to avoid future ptosis. Subcutaneous closure is done with intracutaneous 4-0 Monocryl, which is used to close the superficial layers.

The incision line is covered with tape, and the drains are connected to an evacuation bottle. A sports bra is applied, and an additional supporting strap is fitted on the upper pole of the breast to hold the implant in position.

A perioperative antibiotic is useful in some cases but is not mandatory (in Germany).

Postoperative Care

The patient can remove the tape by herself after 5 days. The sutures are absorbable and do not have to be removed. The drains can be removed if less than 30 ml of drainage is evident in a 24-hour period. This helps prevent hematomas, seromas, and future capsular contracture. A sports bra is worn for 6 weeks, and the supportive strap is worn for 2 weeks. Normal daily activities can be resumed in 8 days.

Follow-Up

The patient receives an implant identification card with all significant information about the surgery and the implants used. The surgeon should register the procedure in a national or an international implant survey. A follow-up visit is recommended 3 months postoperatively and then yearly so changes can be detected promptly.

COMPLICATIONS

Immediate complications include pain, hematoma, and wound infection. To treat pain, ibuprofen is usually sufficient. A hematoma usually will occur within 24 hours of surgery (a 24-hour clinic stay is therefore recommended), and immediate surgical intervention should follow. A compression garment is helpful in cases of rapid filling of the drain when an open vessel lies directly next to the drainage tube; interrupting the vacuum for a few hours is also useful. A wound infection usually requires explantation. A secondary implantation must be delayed for a minimum of 6 to 8 weeks.

Delayed complications include an uncorrectable loss of sensation caused by nerve damage, usually on the lateral border of the breast. A wrong-size implant will usually be revealed when the patient sees her new breasts after the swelling resolves. When this occurs, most patients will ask for a bigger implant. This situation arises when preoperative discussion of implant choices with the patient has been inadequate.

Late complications include incorrect implant positioning, breast deformities, implant rippling, and capsular contracture. Slow upward movement of a subpectoral implant can occur because muscle contracture forces the lower pole of the implant upward. Visible folds and wrinkles on the skin are most often seen with soft, underfilled implants as tissue heals into the textured surfaces and pulls on overlying skin. The implant should be changed in such a case or when a painful contracture of grade 3 or 4 occurs.

CASE STUDIES

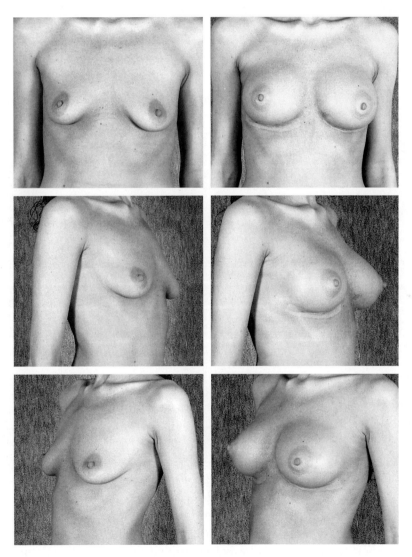

FIG. 7

This 25-year-old woman requested breast augmentation to treat atrophy after pregnancy and breast-feeding. Her breasts were augmented with 320 cc anatomic cohesive gel implants placed through an inframammary incision in the subglandular position. She is shown 3 months postoperatively.

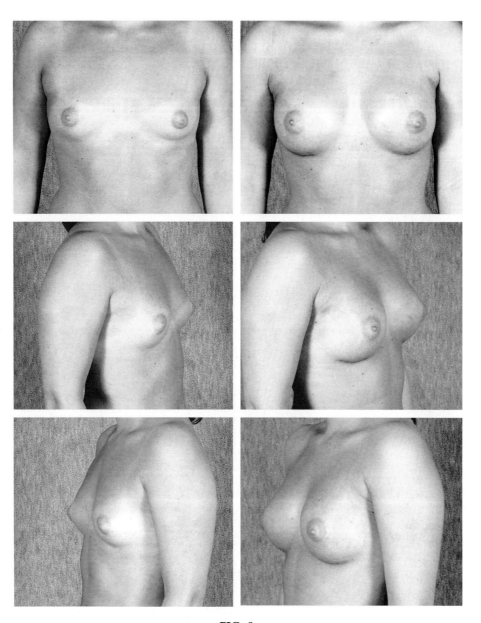

FIG. 8

This young nulliparous woman had micromastia. Her breasts were augmented with 215 cc medium height, anatomic, cohesive gel implants. She is shown 1 month postoperatively.

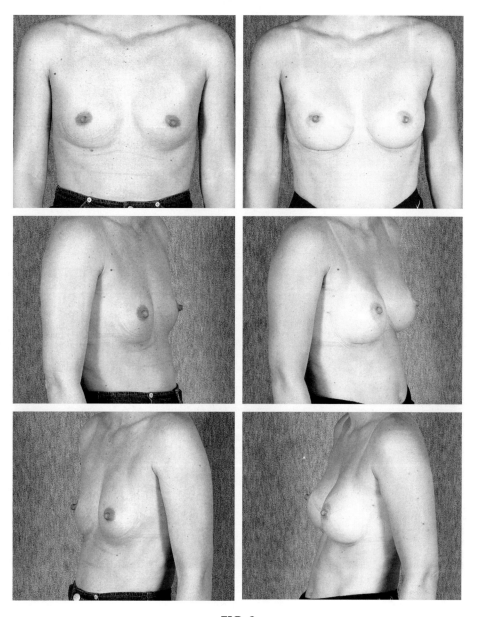

FIG. 9

This 35-year-old woman had micromastia. She had three children but had not breast-fed. Her breasts were augmented with 215 cc anatomic cohesive gel implants. She is shown 3 months postoperatively.

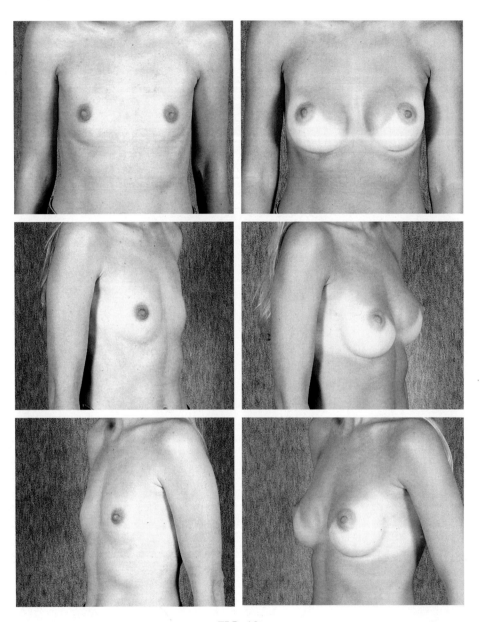

FIG. 10

After one pregnancy and breast-feeding her baby, this 31-year-old patient exhibited signs of micromastia and requested augmentation to achieve larger, fuller breasts. Her breasts were augmented with 245 cc anatomic cohesive gel implants, and she is shown 3 months postoperatively.

The following series of patients demonstrates longer-term follow-up after augmentation using cohesive gel implants. Note how well results have held up over time; the breasts appear soft and symmetrical.

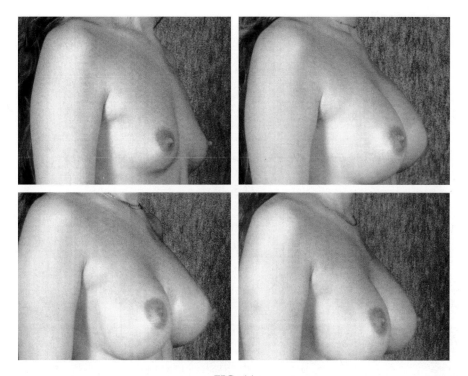

FIG. 11

This patient was 31 years of age when she requested augmentation mammaplasty. Her breasts were augmented with 315 cc cohesive gel implants placed prepectorally. She is shown before surgery and at 5 months, 7 months, and 2 years after surgery.

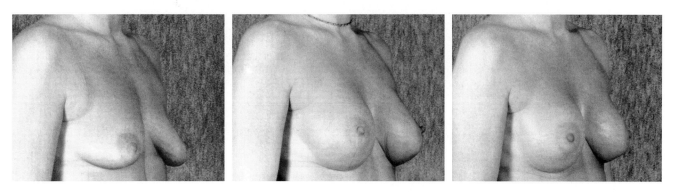

FIG. 12

This 43-year-old patient had bilateral prepectoral augmentation with 280 cc cohesive gel implants. She is shown preoperatively and at 10 months and 4 years postoperatively.

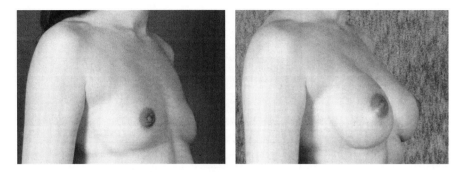

FIG. 13

This patient is shown before and 5 years after augmentation with cohesive gel implants placed prepectorally. She was 35 years old at the time of surgery.

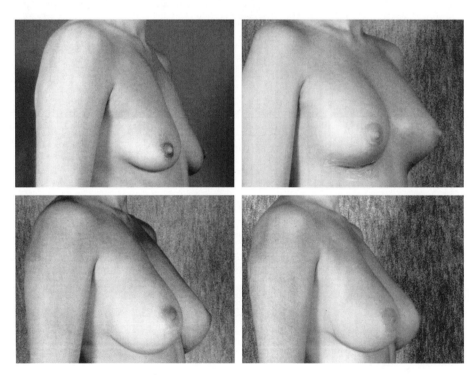

FIG. 14

This 32-year-old patient is shown before breast augmentation and 3 months, 1 year, and 4 years after augmentation with 315 cc implants.

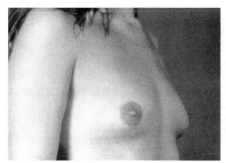 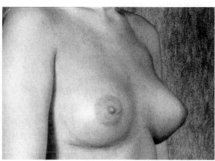 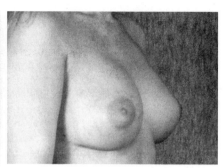

FIG. 15

This 27-year-old patient is shown before breast augmentation and 8 months and 2 years after augmentation with cohesive gel implants placed in a prepectoral position.

SUGGESTED READINGS

Adams WP, Bengston BP, Glicksman CA, et al. Decision and management algorithms to address patient and Food and Drug Administration concerns regarding breast augmentation and implants. Plast Reconstr Surg 114:1252-1257, 2004.

Banbury J, Yetman R, Lucas A, et al. Prospective analysis of the outcome of subpectoral breast augmentation: Sensory changes, muscle function, and body image. Plast Reconstr Surg 113:701-711, 2004.

Brar MI, Tebbetts JB. Early return to normal activities after breast augmentation. Plast Reconstr Surg 110:1193-1195, 2002.

Codner MA, Cohen AT, Hester TR. Complications in breast augmentation: Prevention and correction. Clin Plast Surg 28:587-596, 2001.

Heden P, Jernbeck J, Hober M. Breast augmentation with anatomical cohesive gel implants: The world's largest current experience. Clin Plast Surg 28:531-552, 2001.

Henriksen TF, Holmich LR, Fryzek JP, et al. Incidence and severity of short-term complications after breast augmentation: Results from a nationwide breast implant registry. Ann Plast Surg 51:531-539, 2003.

Hsia HC, Thomson JG. Differences in breast shape preferences between plastic surgeons and patients seeking breast augmentation. Plast Reconstr Surg 112:312-322, 2003.

Karnes J, Morrison W, Salisbury M, et al. Simultaneous breast augmentation and lift. Aesthetic Plast Surg 24:148-154, 2000.

Kompatscher P, Schuler C, Beer GM. The transareolar incision for breast augmentation revisited. Aesthetic Plast Surg 28:70-74, 2004.

Millan Mateo J, Vaquero Perez MM. Innovative new concepts in augmentative breast surgery. Part II: Systematic and drawing. Aesthetic Plast Surg 25:436-442, 2001.

Pleat JM, Dunkin CS, Tyler MP. Communication of risk in breast augmentation. Plast Reconstr Surg 111:2104-2105, 2003.

Ramirez OM, Heller MDL, Tebbetts JB. Dual plane breast augmentation: Avoiding pectoralis major displacement. Plast Reconstr Surg 110:1198-1199, 2002.

Rohrich RJ, Hartley W, Brown S. Incidence of breast and chest wall asymmetry in breast augmentation: A retrospective analysis of 100 patients. Plast Reconstr Surg 111:1513-1523, 2003.

Sarwer DB, La Rossa D, Bartlett SP, et al. Body image concerns of breast augmentation patients. Plast Reconstr Surg 112:83-90, 2003.

Spear SL. Breast augmentation with reduced-height anatomic implants: The pros and cons. Clin Plast Surg 28:561-565, 2001.

Spear SL, Bulan EJ, Venturi ML. Breast augmentation. Plast Reconstr Surg 114:73-81, 2004.

Tebbetts JB. Alternatives and trade-offs in breast augmentation. Clin Plast Surg 28:485-500, 2001.

Tebbetts JB. Breast augmentation with full-height anatomic saline implants: The pros and cons. Clin Plast Surg 28:567-577, 2001.

Tebbetts JB. Does fascia provide additional, meaningful coverage over a breast implant? Plast Reconstr Surg 113:777-780, 2004.

Tebbetts JB. The greatest myths in breast augmentation. Plast Reconstr Surg 107:1895-1903, 2001.

Tebbetts JB. "Out points" criteria for breast implant removal without replacement and criteria to minimize reoperations following breast augmentation. Plast Reconstr Surg 114:1258-1262, 2004.

Tebbetts JB. Pain control in augmentation mammaplasty: The use of indwelling catheters in 200 consecutive patients. Plast Reconstr Surg 113:784-785, 2004.

Tebbetts JB. Patient evaluation, operative planning, and surgical techniques to increase control and reduce morbidity and reoperations in breast augmentation. Clin Plast Surg 28:501-521, 2001.

Tebbetts JB. A surgical perspective from two decades of breast augmentation: Toward state of the art in 2001. Clin Plast Surg 28:425-434, 2001.

Tebbetts JB. A system for breast implant selection based on patient tissue characteristics and implant-soft tissue dynamics. Plast Reconstr Surg Apr 109:1396-1415, 2002.

Tebbetts JB. Warning about a warning about anatomical breast implants. Plast Reconstr Surg 107: 1912-1917, 2001.

Tebbetts JB, Tebbetts TB. An approach that integrates patient education and informed consent in breast augmentation. Plast Reconstr Surg 110:971-981, 2002.

Tofield JJ. Dual plane breast augmentation. Plast Reconstr Surg 108:2162-2164, 2001.

Editorial Commentary

It is interesting how we have come a full circle. In the past almost every implant was placed through an inframammary approach. Then came the transareolar approach, followed by the axillary approach, and, in more recent years, the transumbilical approach. To take the latter first, this seems to fit the American expression, "being a long run for a short slide." I, myself, moved from the periareolar approach to the axillary approach but have, in turn, gone back to the periareolar incision. Certainly the umbilical approach should not be considered for cohesive gel implants, and probably most surgeons have gone for the inframammary approach, which is probably the easiest one to use for this type of more solid implant. The axillary approach can be used, but again is somewhat difficult. Dr. De Lorenzi has very nicely shown that the areolar incision, probably slightly enlarged, allows a cohesive gel implant to be inserted into a submammary or subpectoral position. There is no doubt in my mind that using the areolar approach has been the best for insertion of all implants, whether they be silicone gel or saline-filled. The axillary approach doesn't always result in a good scar, and I believe it is less easy to achieve a good anatomic position with it.

As Professor Olbrisch states, the inframammary incision has been used since the beginnings of breast augmentation surgery, and it should not be disregarded. For many surgeons, it may well be what they consider to be the safest and easiest approach of all. If this results in greater safety for the patient in their hands, then it most certainly should not be dismissed. I certainly feel strongly that, in breast augmentation, the approach to be used is the one that the surgeon is most comfortable with.

Ian T. Jackson, MD

Inframammary fold incisions are very versatile as outlined in this excellent review. The precise location of an inframammary fold incision is sometimes debatable because the skin in this area is sometimes quite mobile, depending on arm position, whether the patient is upright or supine, and the fullness of the breast. The final quality of the scar will be improved if it is made at the correct level on the chest using an appropriate length to prevent tissue maceration during surgery. Postoperatively, if the wound is supported for a prolonged period with plain Micropore Surgical Tape (3M Corporation, St. Paul, MN) (a hypoallergenic paper tape that leaves minimal adhesive residue and is breathable, inexpensive, and minimally irritating to patients). An incision placed slightly too high, so that it ends up on the lower pole of the breast, is much preferable to an incision that is too low on the chest (i.e., below the inframammary fold). The preoperative markings in Figs. 3, 4, and 5 show a dotted line outlining a proposed pocket location that extends above the transverse line across the apexes of the anterior axillary folds. The breast should not in my opinion extend above this line, although in some situations it is necessary to dissect the pocket above this level. Although Professor Olbrisch recommends blunt subpectoral dissection, it is my belief that careful pocket dissection with magnification and electrosurgery to obtain hemostasis is preferable for the patient and the surgeon alike. I agree with Professor Olbrisch that blunt dissection is safe and effective, and that most blood vessels that are avulsed (torn) typically stop bleeding spontaneously and with pressure (as they are apparently designed to do). However, this is not typical of any other plastic surgery technique where we typically pride ourselves in accurate bloodless dissection, and I see no reason why this procedure should be any different. A careful pocket dissection under absolute surgical control will be rewarded with a nice, clean, bloodless pocket that has a lower incidence of postoperative pain and bruising as well as a lower risk of encapsulation (in my opinion, considerable blood in the tissues is a risk factor for capsule formation).

With respect to the amount of pectoralis muscle to release medially, I do not think that the medial border of the pectoralis should be released up to the level of the areola as recommended in the article. If there is some degree of skin laxity, but still some lower pole skin visible in the frontal view (with the patient upright and arms at her side), then some degree of submammary dissection is also required. This releases the breast from the anterior surface of the pectoralis muscle so that the implant can descend in the pocket, preventing a snoopy deformity. The extent of release will depend on the extent of laxity, but it usually does not extend above the nipple. The release of the pectoralis medially should not extend very much above the level of the inframammary crease to prevent breast deformity during pectoralis contraction. I agree with Professor Olbrisch that retromammary placement is superior to retropectoral placement if there is sufficient tissue coverage. If there is insufficient tissue coverage, then retropectoral placement is mandatory.

Extreme care must be taken not to lower the inframammary fold unless it is necessary to do so. In my opinion, the nipple areolar complexes are too high on the breast mounds of the patient shown in Fig. 10. Patients who have constricted breasts have abnormal fold development and require significant manipulation of the inframammary folds, but patients with normal folds should not have them altered unless requesting extreme augmentation that is inappropriate for their anatomy. Instead, it is important for the surgeon to precisely measure the width of the natural breast and select an implant that will fit appropriately. In addition, the patient in Fig. 10 has medial border implant visibility with a recurved portion visible next to the chest wall—the so called "Baywatch breast." Although I have patients who sometimes request this appearance, it is not natural, and in my opinion surgeons should resist providing this. The long-term sequelae of this are tissue thinning and implant visibility. This article is an excellent summary of the surgical technique, postoperative routine, and required aftercare.

Claudio De Lorenzi, BA, MD

Breast Augmentation: Periareolar Approach With Cohesive Gel Implants

Claudio De Lorenzi, BA, MD

Several approaches exist for the successful utilization of cohesive gel breast implants. The most commonly used approach uses an inframammary incision because it affords an excellent view of the implant pocket for hemostasis, allows manipulation of the fascia and the pectoralis, and allows assessment of implant positioning before closure. Periareolar incisions provide similar visual access of the pocket, and hemostasis is theoretically easier because the distance to the furthest area is less than in an inframammary approach.

A periareolar approach to breast augmentation is not new.[1-4] Typically, the technique may be used in any patient requesting augmentation, except when larger devices are planned for patients with smaller areolar diameters, as discussed later. The Montgomery glands help camouflage any irregularity of the incision such as the point where the suture knots are tied.

PATIENT SELECTION

Typically, periareolar incisions are indicated whenever camouflage of the incision is desirable. There is always an underlying concern when patients with dark-pigmented skin present for surgery. However, periareolar incisions typically heal well as long as basic plastic surgery principles are followed. A family history of keloids, hypertrophic scarring, or abnormal wound healing should be noted because these are known risk factors, especially in people with dark-pigmented skin. Because these conditions may indicate a tendency for poor healing and unfavorable scarring, these patients should be offered the option of a more-hidden incision location. The surgeon should do everything possible to minimize the risk of hypertrophic scarring, including gentle tissue handling, sharp incision technique, and minimal blunt tension trauma from retractors and instruments. Rough tissue handling may result in abnormal inflammation and poor healing with postinflammatory hyperpigmentation, especially in patients with dark pigmentation. It is of utmost importance to use an incision sufficient for the proposed implant size. An incision of 5 cm is the recommended minimum for implants that are approximately 250 cc, with larger incisions needed for larger devices. Poor wound healing and unfavorable scarring can be expected when insufficient exposure results in tissue maceration from pulling on the tissues to gain access.

TECHNIQUE
Markings and Incisions

The incision length depends on the diameter of the areola (Fig. 1). An unstretched areolar diameter of 3.5 cm will result in an incision of approximately 5 cm. The patient is marked for augmentation in the upright position, with the arms abducted at the shoulder to simulate the position on the operating table. To attain this position the surgeon may ask the patient to place her hands high on her hips. The edge of the areola is marked at the zone of the last color change. Although the brownish-pink color of the areola sometimes fades indistinctly, especially in nulliparous patients, in most women it is defined clearly. The area should be marked so that the surgeon's blade can stay on the lighter side of the demarcation line. Because a scar will eventually become pale and hypopigmented, it has the best chance of being hidden on the pale side of the line. Creating a dotted line with a surgical marker is a good idea, because the precise location of the color change in the tissues can be seen between the dots during surgery. Loupe magnification adds precision.

The first incision through the dermis should be perpendicular to the surface, but if visible, the underlying muscular tissue should be left on the areolar side of the incision. The subcutaneous fatty tissue is divided, angled away from the nipple-areola complex to avoid undermining it. When the anterior lamella of Scarpa's fascia is encountered, the fascia can be used as a plane of dissection down to the prepectoral fascia. Usually the lower border of the pectoralis major muscle is dissected even if a submammary approach is planned. Once the lower border of the pectoralis muscle is visible, the external oblique, rectus abdominis, and serratus anterior muscles may be visible in the area immediately adjacent to it. Occasionally when performing a subfascial dissection (or any form of submammary dissection), the sternalis muscle is found.[5] The presence of this muscle is variable; it may be found on the medial aspect of the chest, sometimes bilaterally, adjacent to the sternum. Its fibers extend vertically from the manubrium to the sixth or seventh costal cartilage, and it occupies the space above the medial part of the

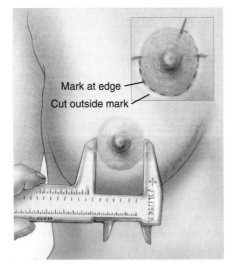

Mark at edge
Cut outside mark

FIG. 1   Marking for a periareolar incision is made at the junction of the area of the color change from the pink of the areola to the color of the skin. A dotted line helps the surgeon see the color change while making the incision.

pectoralis major muscle, detectable in approximately 4% of the population.[6] It is important only because it may be mistaken for a pathologic condition. Note that it also may appear on mammograms at the approximate depth of the medial nodes.

Plane of Dissection

Typically dissection is performed either under the fascia or under the pectoralis major muscle (Fig. 2). There are advantages to a prepectoral plane of dissection. The submammary plane (meaning subfascial) has the advantage of not having abnormal dynamics during patient muscular activity. When using the periareolar approach, the central part of the fascia may be left in place (Fig. 3). This is not an avascular plane; numerous small

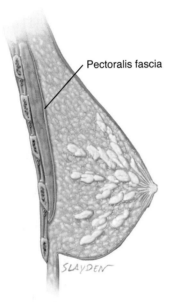

FIG. 2   The pectoralis fascia firmly adheres to the pectoralis major muscle. Multiple vascular fibrous bands join the fascia to the underlying muscle fibers. Although the fascia itself is thin, its adherence to the muscle helps reduce implant edge visibility.

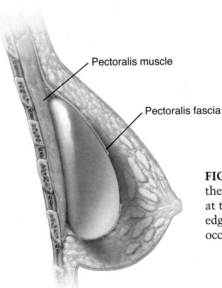

FIG. 3   Subfascial implant placement. Note how the edge of the pectoralis muscle is pulled up slightly at the implant edge. This helps mask the implant edge and prevent undermining, which sometimes occurs with submammary placement.

bleeding vessels will be encountered. The surgeon should use traditional scissor dissection with cautery of the bleeding vessels or electrosurgical techniques. Using needle point cautery and smoke evacuation, the fascia may be elevated precisely from the underlying muscle, but this is sometimes difficult because of muscle contraction. The muscle is treated as gently as possible, and electrosurgery is used with precision to prevent subsequent discomfort and to minimize fulguration of normal tissues. Using a fine needle point reduces the amount of tissue damage. This is important because burned tissue will cause internal scarring as well as a postoperative serous fluid effusion; it may also promote capsule formation. Precise dissection with minimal blood "staining" of tissues is ideal and may reduce the risk of capsule contraction. Several vertical segments of tissue are encountered deep to the fascia that fix the fascia firmly to the underlying muscular bundles. These may be quite vascular and may be treated with bipolar electrosurgery instead of monopolar electrosurgery, because this also reduces the amount of tissue injury. A fiberoptic, lighted retractor is of great assistance in the dissection to permit a clear view, and it is helpful to have an assistant to help retract. The dissection must proceed carefully, taking into account the size of the implant to be used.

When placing cohesive gel implants, the size of the pocket must not greatly exceed that of the implant, unlike saline implants, which require larger pockets. However, it is critical that the pocket be made large enough to accommodate the implant. If there must be any error, one should err by making the pocket slightly smaller. Although it is possible to slightly enlarge the pocket with the implant in place, it is preferable to make it the correct size before implant insertion. For example, a Mentor Contour Profile Gel (CPG) Medium 280 cc implant is 12 cm wide, but only 11.3 cm tall, and the pocket dimensions must match the ratio. A pocket that is too narrow will tend to force this type of device to rotate. After insertion, the implant should lie flat without wrinkles. This is especially important with the Biocell Surface (McGhan) device, which has a more aggressive texture. Application of external compression on the breast will help reveal any pocket asymmetry or any areas that are not properly released at the periphery of the augmented breast. If these areas are not readily accessible with retractors through the wound, then the implant should be removed and the pocket enlarged appropriately.

Hemostasis and Irrigation

Complete hemostasis is attained with electrosurgery. Subfascial dissection takes longer than subpectoral pocket dissection, because the subfascial plane is not areolar. An ideal dissection will have little or no staining of soft tissues with blood and a completely dry pocket. In some cases a drain may be advisable, although most of the time I do not use a drain unless performing a complete capsulectomy or another ancillary procedure. The pocket is irrigated several times with normal saline solution. I typically use one syringe of povidone-iodine (Betadine) solution followed by irrigation with normal saline solution until the wash is clear.

Implant Insertion

Before implant insertion, the surgeon prepares the area again and changes gloves. Implants are handled only by the surgeon, who has not touched anything other than the implant and its sterile container. Specifically, no contact is allowed with any cotton, paper products, or anything that might reasonably be expected to have fibers on it. It is my unproven conviction that wood fibers or cotton fibers may be another risk factor for capsular contracture, along with blood and other well-known risk factors. The implant is handled minimally while the surgeon does a quality inspection, then it is inserted through the incision, which is held open by an assistant. Although there may appear to be a significant size discrepancy between the size of the implant and the size of the opening, this can be overcome. With practice even those who have never seen it done learn how to manipulate the implant until it is eased into the pocket. It is a good idea for a novice to practice with a sizer or sample beforehand. A rigid towel mounted on a frame with an appropriately sized opening cut into it will help the novice learn to manipulate the devices.

After placing the implant it is important to use a blunt instrument such as a large dilator to redrape breast tissue over the implant evenly and to ensure there are no folds on the implant. If there are folds they must be addressed intraoperatively. Folds caused by compression from an inadequate pocket size must be eliminated by enlarging the pocket. If the pocket is large enough, the folds are usually caused by improper positioning and will disappear when the tissues are redraped properly.

Once the implant is in place, the deepest layer of the incision is approximated if possible, especially in patients with firm parenchyma, to prevent herniation of the implant into the incision. Absorbable monofilament sutures are preferred, and only one or two deep sutures are required. One must be very cautious and use utmost care to prevent damage to the device during closure, because losing control of the needle may result in perforation during placement of the deep sutures. It is helpful to have an assistant retract the edges of the opening. Closure is done in layers, starting with the deepest layer next to the implant (taking utmost care to avoid puncturing the implant), then the deep subdermal fibrofatty tissues, and finally the deep dermis. The final closure is made with half-buried horizontal mattress sutures at either end of a running subcuticular closure; the knot scar will mimic a Montgomery gland and be less noticeable.

COMPLICATIONS
Hypertrophic Scars

Prevention of hypertrophic scars is best; this may be accomplished by using a good surgical technique with minimal tissue maceration, gentle tissue handling, and precise wound closure. Risk of hypertrophic scars may also be reduced by applying long-term support of the incision with paper tape. The tape is worn constantly, and patients are instructed to change the tape only when it begins to fall off, typically once every week or so. Patients may shower with the tape in place. If patients develop sensitivity to the tape, then other types of gentle compression such as silicone gel sheeting may be effective. However, cleanliness is difficult with occlusive dressings of this nature. In rare cases injections of triamcinolone (Kenalog) may be required. I begin with a dilution of 5 mg triamcinolone per cc. Kenalog comes in a strength of 40 mg per cc, and if injected at full strength, it may cause severe tissue atrophy. However, some patients do require larger doses, and I assess the patient's response at 14 days. If there is not a good response, I double the strength of the triamcinolone to 10 mg per cc. If there is still no response after another 14 days, I double the strength again to 20 mg per cc. It is important to titrate the dose to the response, because tissue atrophy and telangiectasia may occur in sensitive patients that may take months or years to resolve. The solution must be injected directly into the hypertrophic scar tissue. Scar tissue is usually dense, so the amount of fluid that can be injected directly into it is quite modest. Ice applied topically for a few moments before injection may help reduce the initial discomfort and subsequent bruising. Inject a small area first and wait a few moments to allow the local anesthetic in the solution to work. The remainder of the treatment should proceed from anesthetized toward nonanesthetized skin, so that the patient should really only have to suffer one needle injection through the skin during any one treatment session. This technique should become easier, and the patient should be less tender during subsequent sessions.

Loss of Nipple Sensitivity

Loss of nipple sensitivity is uncommon with this technique, occurring in less than 5% of cases. In fact, my clinical impression is that loss of nipple sensation is more related to implant size than incision placement. Larger implants likely are related to loss of nipple sensation, similar to any other technique of breast augmentation. Other complications are similar to those encountered with other techniques of breast augmentation.

Approximately 50% of 400 cases have been performed using the periareolar approach with good results and few hypertrophic scars or other complications requiring revision. Two patients with dark pigmentation required further wound management; one patient of Mediterranean extraction required a late scar revision; and one patient with a history of hypertrophic scarring developed hypertrophic scarring in spite of maximum wound care. It resolved with compression and triamcinolone injections.

RESULTS

The patient shown in Fig. 4 was 39 years old with two children, and was 5 feet, 4 inches tall and 114 pounds before surgery (A, C, and E). She was treated with a 245 cc Mentor Medium CPG implant in the subfascial space. She underwent uneventful subfascial augmentation using a periareolar technique. She is shown at the completion of surgery immediately before a tape bandage was applied (G). Her postoperative course was uneventful. She is shown 3 years postoperatively (B, D, and F). The scars are well healed with minimal visibility: H, left breast; and I, right breast after 3 years. The breast implants are soft and in good position, and no abnormalities are present.

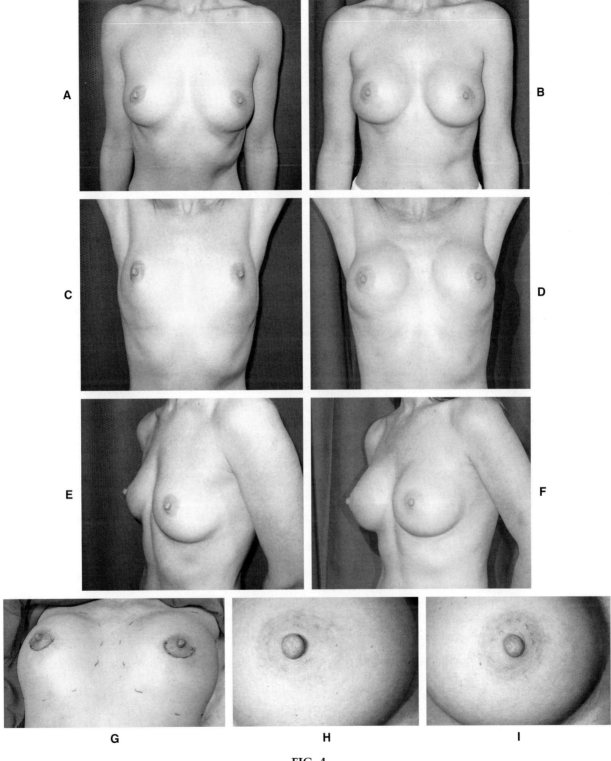

FIG. 4

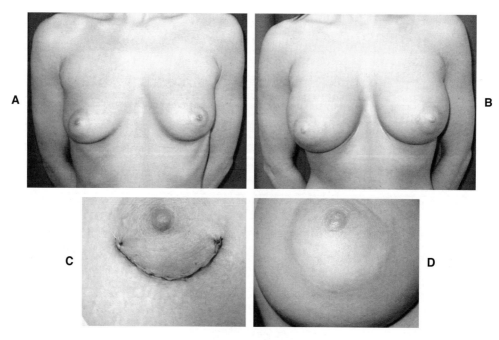

FIG. 5

This 25-year-old patient was nulliparous, was 5 feet, 6 inches tall, and weighed 122 pounds. *A* and *B,* Her breasts were augmented with 315 cc Mentor Medium CPG devices through periareolar incisions. She is shown preoperatively and 18 months postoperatively. The close-up views show standard closure before bandage application *(C)* and a follow-up view of the scar at 18 months *(D).*

REFERENCES

1. McKinney P, Shedbalker AR. Augmentation mammaplasty using a non-inflatable prosthesis through a circum-areolar incision. Br J Plast Surg 27:35-38, 1974.
2. Jones FR, Tauras AP. A periareolar incision for augmentation mammaplasty. Plast Reconstr Surg 51:641-644, 1973.
3. Norman JD, Snyder GB. Augmentation mammaplasty through a circumareolar incision using a solid, gel-filled implant. South Med J 68:1456-1457, 1975.
4. Spear SL, Matsuba H, Little JW III. The medial periareolar approach to submuscular augmentation mammaplasty under local anesthesia. Plast Reconstr Surg 84:599-606, 1989.
5. Harish K, Gopinath KS. Sternalis muscle: Importance in surgery of the breast. Surg Radiol Anat 25:311-314, 2003.
6. Saeed M, Murshid KR, Rufai AA, et al. Sternalis. An anatomic variant of chest wall musculature. Saudi Med J 23:1214-1221, 2002.

Editorial Commentary

Dr. De Lorenzi speaks from a great deal of experience using cohesive gel implants. He has placed these implants in 400 patients, and half of these have been placed using the periareolar approach.

Our experience using the periareolar approach with standard gel-filled implants has been a very happy one, but of course insertion is much easier in average patients. However, there are patients who want very large implants placed through very short periareolar incisions, and, as described in this article, these cases simply require good retraction and careful technique. In my own experience, beginning with using submammary incisions in the dim and distant past followed by periareolar incisions and then going enthusiastically into the axillary approach, my nurses and myself all quickly realized that the periareolar approach gave as good an exposure as any of the others, but there was a learning curve. However, the important things are that this technique really provides the least obvious scars and, if performed properly, is virtually problem-free. Obviously, with gel-filled implants in general, and with cohesive gel implants in particular, there is apprehension about using what seems to be a more limited approach. But when one tries it and follows the instructions given in this article, it easily becomes one's favorite method of placing gel-filled breast implants of any type.

Another important feature of this article is the advice about the very careful handling of the implants and the careful closure of the wound. These instructions are virtually mandatory, and deviating from them will result in grief. I heartily concur with Dr. De Lorenzi that loss of nipple sensation is extremely rare.

In conclusion, the periareolar approach is safe, simple, and in my experience, almost complication-free.

Ian T. Jackson, MD

Breast Reconstruction

Maurizio Nava, MD; Andrea Spano, MD; Angela Pennati, MD;
Umberto Cortinovis, MD; Stefano Bonomi, MD; Phillip Blondeel, MD, PhD

Breast reconstruction using textured implant devices filled with highly cohesive silicone gel is effective for both immediate and delayed reconstruction following mastectomy. Reproducing breast projection and recreating the inframammary fold are the greatest technical challenges of reconstructing the breast, and biodimensional cohesive gel prostheses are capable of achieving good projection and ptosis.

HISTORY

In 1963 mammary prostheses became commercially available as rounded devices filled with silicone gel, and saline-filled implants were launched a few years later in 1965. The Becker permanent expander (Mentor, Santa Barbara, CA) has been in use for almost 2 decades and has the advantage of permitting gradual tissue expansion without a need for subsequent replacement. The round Becker implant has historically been the most popular round prosthesis for breast reconstruction even though it has some shortcomings such as a limited ability to expand the lower portion of the breast, a possibility of subcutaneous rippling (most evident in the upper quadrants), and a lack of a natural ptotic shape. However today, with the introduction of the contoured-shaped Becker expander implant, these problems have been overcome. To address the most difficult aspects of breast reconstruction such as creating a natural breast contour, textured, anatomic implant designs were introduced (Fig. 1).

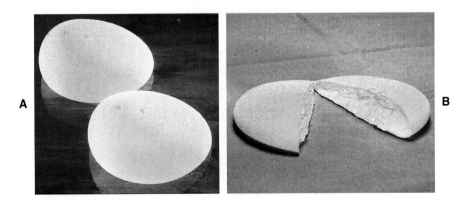

FIG. 1 **A,** Anatomic, textured implants filled with highly cohesive silicone gel. **B,** A textured implant filled with highly cohesive silicone gel shows no silicone leakage after being ruptured.

During the past decade, breast reconstruction techniques have focused on contour rather than just volume replacement. Anatomically shaped devices can be used with these techniques for both one-stage and two-stage procedures. Single-stage reconstruction with implants is an option only for some patients. For all other cases two-stage implant reconstruction may provide a more natural appearance than using an implant alone. If a mastectomy has been performed previously, a two-stage delayed reconstruction should take place.

TIMING OF BREAST RECONSTRUCTION
Immediate Reconstruction

Immediate breast reconstruction should be offered to most patients undergoing mastectomy. It does not affect the chances of carcinoma recurrence, and it does not make detection of local carcinoma recurrence more difficult. Many factors influence the choice of using autologous tissue or implants for reconstruction; the most important factors to consider are chemotherapy and chest wall irradiation. Chemotherapy can be started after the mastectomy wounds are healed, although there is inevitably an increased risk of septic complications that might necessitate removing an implant. Autologous reconstruction is a good choice for immediate reconstruction when postoperative chest wall irradiation is planned. Other factors influencing the decision to use autologous tissue or an implant are the age and physical status of the patient. Immediate prosthesis insertion avoids additional costs of further hospitalization, and reconstruction using an implant adds only 60 to 90 minutes to the operating time. Immediate breast reconstruction benefits patients psychologically and improves their quality of life. A poor prognosis in itself is not a contraindication to breast reconstruction, although reconstruction should be undertaken cautiously in patients considered to be at a particularly high risk for local recurrence.

Delayed Reconstruction

The primary indication for delayed breast reconstruction is a previous mastectomy. The requirements for successful reconstruction in this context are generally more rigorous than those for immediate reconstruction. The patient's oncologic status should be confirmed before discussing reconstruction to ensure there is no evidence of local or distant disease recurrence. The tissues of the chest wall must be carefully examined, giving attention to the quality of skin, scars, and the pectoralis major muscle. If the chest wall musculature is severely atrophic and associated with thin, tight skin, implant insertion is contraindicated. Previous chest wall irradiation is not an absolute contraindication for using an implant, but the risk of ischemic complications indicates that an autologous reconstruction may be preferable. Large breasts are a relative contraindication to implant reconstruction because of volume limitations using tissue expansion techniques.

INDICATIONS FOR IMPLANT RECONSTRUCTION
One-Stage Reconstruction

One-stage reconstruction is suitable for patients with small breasts and minimal ptosis, because a permanent cohesive gel–filled prosthesis can be inserted without preliminary tissue expansion. Anatomic, textured implants filled with highly cohesive silicone gel have enhanced durability, reduced incidence of capsule formation, and less tendency to migrate within the chest wall; they also have less tendency for gravity to pull the con-

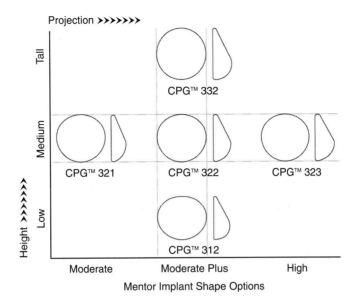

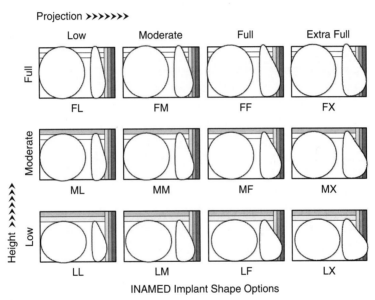

FIG. 2   Anatomic, textured implants filled with highly cohesive silicone gel are available in a variety of shapes.

tents of the implant into the lower pole than implants filled with noncohesive gel or saline. Innovations in the design of textured implants filled with highly cohesive silicone gel emphasize breast shape and permit reconstruction of breasts with a more natural feel and appearance. These implants are available in a broad range of specifications for base width, height, and projection (Fig. 2).

Because of the variety of options offered, implants can be tailored to each patient, and surgeons can precisely plan a three-dimensional reconstruction. Matching a reconstructed breast to the contralateral breast is also easier when there are a number of implant sizes to choose from. Newer techniques permit breast reconstruction increasingly based on aesthetic considerations and the expectations of patients. The one-stage reconstruction procedure, even for a medium-large breast, can be completed using a new technique called a skin reducing mastectomy.

Two-Stage Reconstruction

Two-stage reconstruction is appropriate for patients with medium to ptotic breasts. The use of temporary expanders with complementary permanent prostheses has greatly advanced the field of prosthetic breast reconstruction. Anatomic, textured expanders permit rapid expansion with lower pressures in the implant. Compared with round and smooth implants, they are less likely to migrate and result in a chest wall deformity. It is also easy to achieve a good inframammary fold with lower pole definition. Most devices have an integral injection port that does not require an additional procedure for removal. Expandable, saline-filled gel implants have been developed to provide more natural projection and give improved contour to the upper breast. Following tissue expansion, the tissue expander must be replaced with a cohesive gel–filled prosthesis.

PREOPERATIVE PLANNING
Mastectomy

A modified radical mastectomy preserves the mammary skin envelope and the underlying subcutaneous tissue. The nipple-areola complex (usually with a surrounding ellipse of skin) is removed, along with the glandular tissue and the fascial attachments of the breast.

From a reconstructive point of view, certain anatomic features are critical for optimal results:

1. Preservation of the inframammary fold frame
2. Integrity of the pectoralis major muscle
3. Quality and tension of the skin flaps
4. Preservation of the nipple-areola complex (if a nipple-sparing mastectomy can be performed adequately and there are no oncological contraindications)

For cases in which the inframammary fold must be sacrificed, a new fold can be fashioned at the time of reconstruction or during subsequent surgery for implant revision. There must be sufficient skin to allow primary closure without tension following insertion of the implant. When a tissue expander is used, it is inflated minimally at the time of initial placement to avoid excessive tension on the skin, subcutaneous tissues, or pectoral muscles. The upper mastectomy flap can be undermined superiorly if necessary, but it is preferable to avoid dissection of the lower flap beyond the inframammary fold.

It is unnecessary to remove the fascia over the pectoralis major muscle, although this structure should be excised if a tumor is attached. The pectoralis major and serratus anterior muscles are preserved, whereas the pectoralis minor can be excised or divided to facilitate access to level III nodes lying medial to the muscle. If a skin-sparing mastectomy is performed, the skin of the breast is preserved except for the nipple-areola complex, and there will be an opportunity to perform a one-stage reconstruction or a two-stage, short-term expansion procedure. If a nipple-sparing mastectomy can be performed, there will be no need to reconstruct the nipple-areola complex after breast reconstruction.

Design

It is important to plan the operation using a geometric approach; the overall shape and contour of the new breast will relate to three parameters: width, height, and projection (Fig. 3). The patient should stand in front of the surgeon with her hands on her flanks while the preoperative markings are carefully planned (Fig. 4).

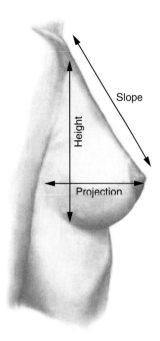

FIG. 3   Three-dimensional shape of the breast.

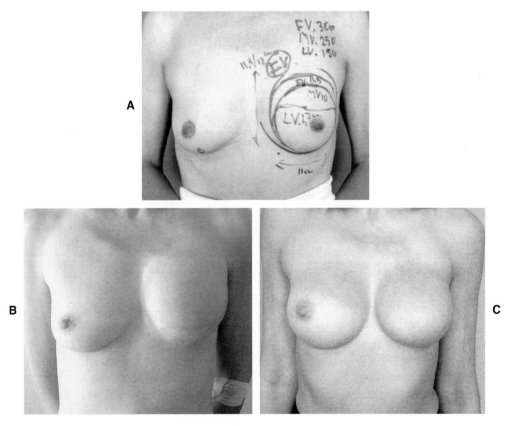

FIG. 4   First-stage immediate reconstruction (expander insertion). **A,** Preoperative markings. **B,** Before expander removal and contralateral augmentation. **C,** 1-year follow-up.

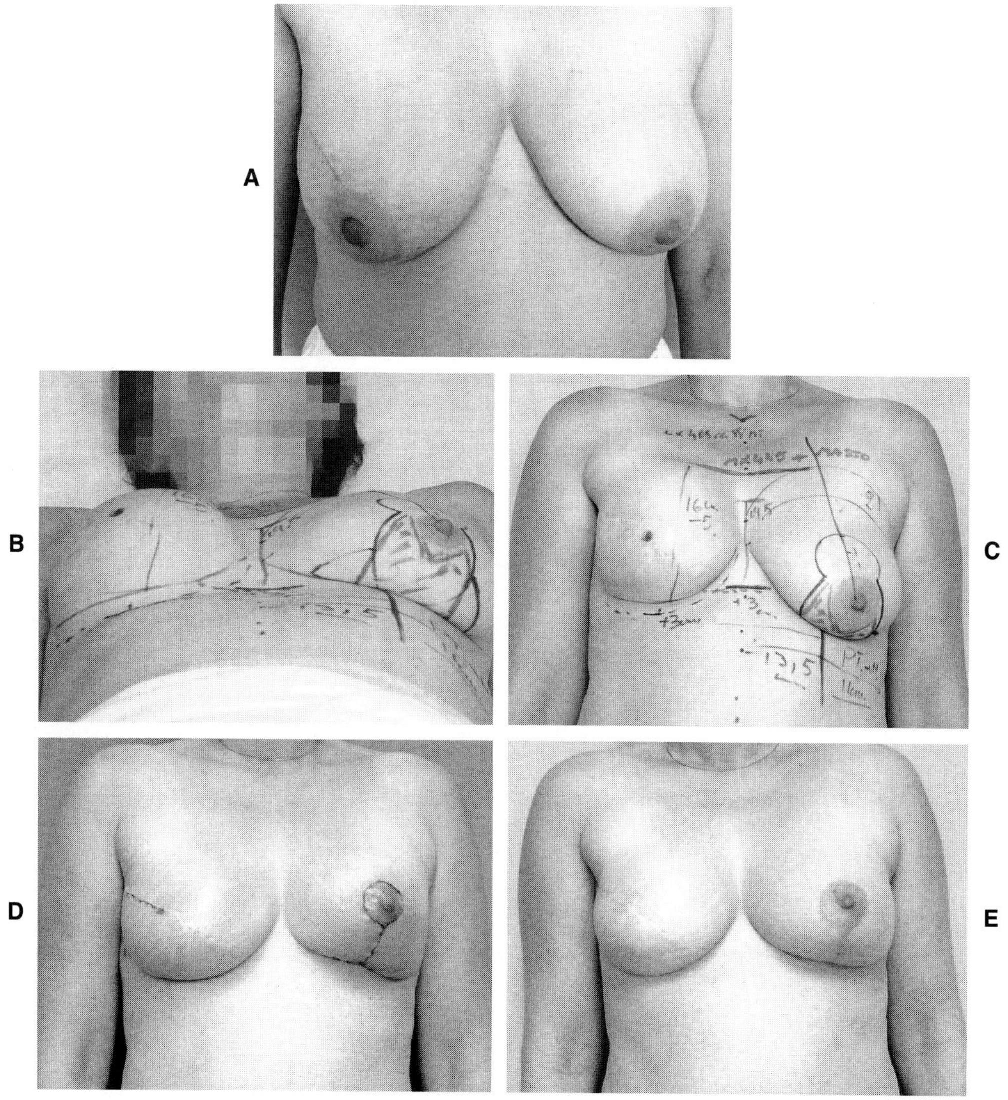

FIG. 5   Second-stage immediate reconstruction (implant insertion) and contralateral mastopexy.
A, Preoperatively. **B** and **C,** Markings for expander removal and contralateral mastopexy. **D,** Postoperative result. **E,** 9-month follow-up.

Base width and height are determined by the dimensions of the contralateral breast and are measured out on the chest wall corresponding precisely to the site of implant insertion (Figs. 5 and 6).

The projection of the breast can be predicted to some extent from the dimensions of the implant, although the final result will only be apparent once expansion has occurred. Depending on the final volume of inflation, a permanent anatomic prosthesis can be selected that has an appropriate width, height, and projection. The most important measurement is the width. An appropriate height and projection will be determined based on the health of the breast and the patient's wishes. The surgeon must be able to think in three dimensions when planning breast reconstruction.

If an expander will be used, the surface markings of the subpectoral pocket can be outlined on the chest wall using the manufacturer's templates to select a low-, medium-,

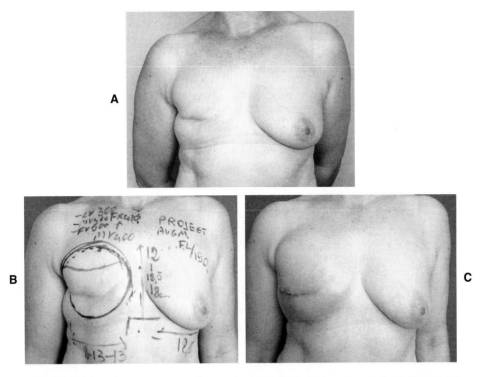

FIG. 6 First-stage delayed reconstruction (expander insertion). **A,** Preoperatively. **B,** Preoperative markings. **C,** Postoperative result.

or full-shape expandable prosthesis. When the opposite breast is very large or will be augmented, then an expander one size bigger should be chosen.

The lower border of the pocket should lie just at the level of the submammary crease. The submuscular pocket will have the same dimensions as the selected expander and will reflect the base width and height of the contralateral breast. However, for delayed reconstruction, very large expanders should be avoided because they may be incompatible with chest wall dimensions. A template is positioned on the chest wall in line with the inframammary crease (Fig. 6).

The final expander volume after inflation should correspond to its capacity, and the expander may be overfilled if necessary. Ideally, the final volume adjustment should be carried out only after any contralateral surgery is performed and the final size of the reconstructed breast can be determined intraoperatively.

OPERATIVE TECHNIQUE
One-Stage Breast Reconstruction
Intraoperative Planning

The patient must be correctly positioned on the operating table. Though initially in the supine position, the patient's position will be changed after mastectomy and before final reconstruction. The patient's arms should lie at an angle of 60 degrees to the body on the operating table, thus completely relaxing the pectoralis major muscle and facilitating blunt dissection of the submuscular pocket. The contralateral breast should be exposed because it is a useful guide to form the subpectoral pocket and determine the appropriate position of the inframammary fold.

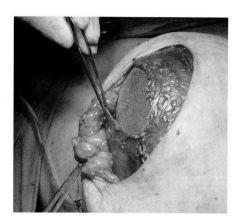

FIG. 7 The serratus muscle is used to cover the lateral border of the implant.

Surgical Steps

1. Preparation of a submuscular pocket. The mastectomy incision should be chosen with input from the oncologist who is performing the breast ablation. The serratus muscle or the serratus fascia, if well represented, is dissected to cover the lateral part of the implant (Fig. 7). From the lateral border of the pectoralis major muscle dissection is performed beneath the pectoralis major muscle superiorly, medially, and inferiorly. Then the sternal attachments of the pectoralis major are dissected from the second intercostal space to the inferior edge of the pocket. Finally, the lowermost attachments of the pectoralis major and the serratus anterior muscles are dissected at the level of the contralateral inframammary fold. The pocket ideally should be completely submuscular, except at the inframammary fold where it should extend into the deep fascial layer, avoiding direct continuity with the mastectomy site.
2. Insertion of two suction drains. Drains should be placed in the submuscular pocket and axilla following axillary dissection.
3. Insertion of the correctly oriented prosthesis. Attention should be paid to filling the lower pole of the breast.
4. Closure of the muscular pocket. Interrupted sutures can be inserted before placement of the prosthesis to minimize the risk of needle puncture.
5. Closure of subcutaneous tissues and skin.

Two-Stage Breast Reconstruction: Immediate
Intraoperative Planning for Insertion of Expander (First Stage)

The position of the patient is the same as described previously for one-stage breast reconstruction.

Surgical Steps

1. Preparation of a submuscular pocket. An incision is made along the lateral border of the pectoralis major muscle. Progressive dissection is performed beneath the pectoralis major muscle superiorly, medially, and inferiorly. The inferior part of the dissection can include the anterior rectus sheath and the aponeurosis of the external oblique muscle and continue beneath the serratus anterior muscle. Then the sternal attachments of the pectoralis major are dissected from the second intercostal space to the inferior edge of the pocket, and the lowermost attachments of the pectoralis

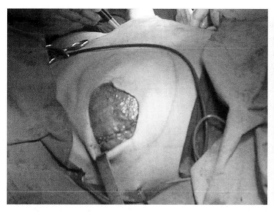 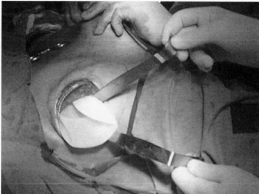

FIG. 8   Expander insertion.

major and the serratus anterior muscle are dissected at the level of the contralateral inframammary fold. Ideally the pocket should be completely submuscular, except at the inframammary fold where it should extend into the deep fascial layer, avoiding direct continuity with the mastectomy site.

2. Preparation of the expander. Any air in the inner expansion chamber of the expander must be completely evacuated. The expander is partially inflated with saline to ensure there is no leakage. A small amount of saline (up to 20% final volume) is left within the prosthesis because partial inflation will aid insertion. Then the prosthesis is immersed in povidone iodine solution.
3. Insertion of two suction drains. Drains should be placed in the submuscular pocket and axilla following axillary dissection.
4. Insertion of the partially inflated and correctly oriented prosthesis. Attention should be paid to filling the lower pole of the breast (Fig. 8).
5. Closure of the submuscular pocket. Interrupted sutures can be inserted before placement of the prosthesis to minimize the risk of needle puncture.
6. Closure of subcutaneous tissues and skin.
7. Inflation of the expander. The expander is inflated with 200 to 300 ml of saline. Initial expansion is desirable provided there is no skin tension.

Two-Stage Breast Reconstruction: Delayed
Intraoperative Planning for Insertion of Expander (First Stage)

The patient is positioned on the table supine with her arms out on a board, and the level of the inframammary fold is marked. The surgeon checks the chosen expander size in relation to the thorax and the contralateral breast. The volume and shape of the latter can be modified at the time of reconstruction, which demands careful planning involving both patient and surgeon.

Surgical Steps

1. Skin incision. The incision is placed toward the upper lateral portion of the mastectomy scar. The pectoralis major muscle is incised either along its free lateral edge, or more centrally along the line of the muscle fibers.

2. Preparation of the submuscular pocket. Progressive dissection is performed deep to the pectoralis major muscle superiorly, medially, and inferiorly. The medial and low-ermost attachments of the pectoralis major are dissected from the level of the fourth rib to the level of the sixth and seventh ribs. Any constricted scar tissue in the infra-mammary region is excised.

The remaining steps are similar to those described previously for immediate implant reconstruction. The wound is closed with absorbable sutures.

Breast Reconstruction After Expansion (Second Stage)

The second stage of reconstruction is identical for immediate and delayed procedures and should be undertaken at least 6 months after final expander inflation. The delay allows for stabilization and improves the potential ptosis achievable with expansion. In this stage, the temporary tissue expander is removed and is replaced with a permanent implant. Furthermore, minor refinements can be made to the reconstructed breast such as enlarging the pocket and contouring the breast. Experience is required for choosing an appropriate size and shape of prosthesis, but using textured implants filled with highly cohesive silicone gel makes this selection process easier.

INTRAOPERATIVE PLANNING FOR PROSTHESIS INSERTION

The results of previous augmentation, reduction, or mastopexy procedures modify the surgical approach to the final postmastectomy reconstruction. Both breasts should be visible in the operative field, and the level of the contralateral inframammary fold should be marked.

SURGICAL STEPS

1. Skin incision. To remove the expander, the skin incision is placed toward the lateral end of the postmastectomy scar, and an incision is made either along the free edge of the pectoralis major muscle, or in the line of its muscle fibers.
2. Removal of the temporary tissue expander (Fig. 9).
3. Preparation of the pocket. A pocket is prepared for the final prosthesis using a complete capsulectomy. A complete capsulectomy, except for the aspect that extends onto the thoracic wall, allows a better distribution of the expanded skin over the implant. Extending the lower pole of the new breast is accomplished using a combination of radial and transverse scoring.
4. Creation of the inframammary fold (Fig. 10). Following capsulectomy, the superficial fascia is divided at the level of the inframammary fold, which is marked by needles inserted through the skin into the pouch. The lower edge of the superficial fascia is sutured to the chest wall musculature with continuous sutures of a strong absorbable material (1/0 sutures).
5. Insertion of drains.
6. Insertion of the permanent prosthesis (Fig. 11). Following insertion of the prosthesis, it is important to check the final result by elevating the patient to a sitting position.
7. Closure of the wound. The wound is closed in two layers using soluble suture material.

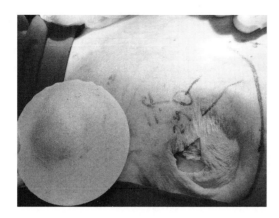

FIG. 9 Expander removal.

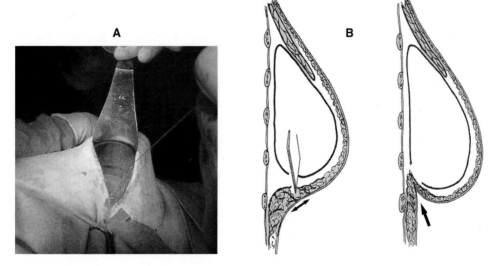

FIG. 10   **A,** Creating a new inframammary fold. **B,** Technique for defining the inframammary fold.

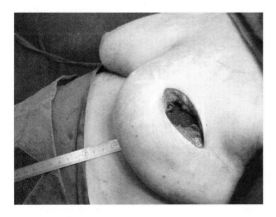

FIG. 11   Replacement of expander with a permanent, anatomic implant filled with highly cohesive silicone gel.

POSTOPERATIVE CARE

Prophylactic antibiotics are administered to avoid staphylococcal infection. Compared with a transverse rectus abdominis muscle (TRAM) flap or a deep inferior epigastric perforator (DIEP) flap, postoperative pain and discomfort is generally of short duration using the procedure described here and can be controlled with routine analgesia. Drains are removed when daily volumes are less than 30 to 40 ml. The mean duration of the hospital stay is less than 5 days with immediate reconstruction and 2 to 4 days with delayed reconstruction. A short period of hospitalization is required when exchanging a temporary implant with a permanent one. Applying bandages can help enhance the inframammary fold, but only surgical correction will create a durable fold. A well-fitting sports bra should be worn following reconstruction and contralateral mastopexy or reduction. Intensive exercise should be avoided for 2 to 3 weeks, although arm and shoulder mobilization is important following formal axillary dissection. Inflation of the prosthesis should be carried out weekly, ideally in a designated outpatient area. The rate of inflation is governed by patient comfort; excessive expansion can produce local pain and discomfort. Expansion takes place over 4 to 8 weeks, and a temporary tissue expander should not be replaced with a permanent implant within 6 months. This allows time for the tissues to adapt and for capsule formation to stabilize. Furthermore, tissues in the lower pole of the breast are stretched by gravitational forces.

COMPLICATIONS

Immediate complications are hematoma formation, skin necrosis, and pain. Adjuvant therapies, including chemotherapy and radiotherapy, can delay wound healing and postpone any planned program of expansion. Later complications include infection, implant extrusion, and capsular contracture. Complications are generally more common with immediate reconstruction than with delayed reconstruction when adjuvant treatments are performed around the time of immediate reconstruction. High-dose chemotherapy can compromise the immune system and influence healing processes. Radiotherapy impairs the ability of the skin to act as a natural barrier to exogenous insults. Irradiation induces excessive fibrosis and reduces tissue oxygen levels, thus promoting excessive capsular reaction. Pressure sores can develop in the lower pole of the breast when the skin is damaged by radiation.

Persistent infection around the implant mandates removal, and further reconstruction attempts must be deferred until the infection resolves and the wound is completely healed. A partially extruded implant must be removed. The degree of capsular contracture after breast reconstruction is generally greater than that occurring following augmentation. When capsule formation leads to constriction or pain, open capsulotomy is required, sometimes with implant exchange. Infection and capsular contracture are relatively uncommon, but secondary procedures to achieve breast symmetry and optimal shape are often necessary.

RESULTS

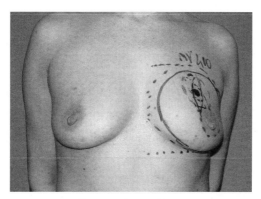

Preoperative markings

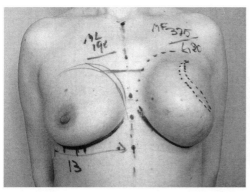

Final implant and contralateral augmentation markings

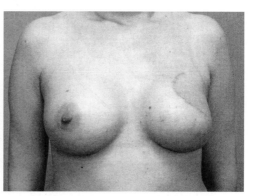

Immediately after surgery

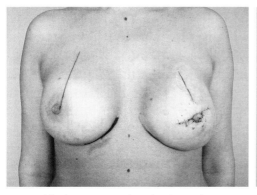

Nipple reconstruction after 6 months

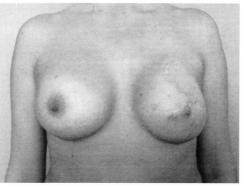

1 year postoperatively

FIG. 12

This 42-year-old patient had a simple left mastectomy for ductal carcinoma in situ (DCIS). At the time of her mastectomy a two-stage immediate reconstruction was begun. Considering the small size of her left breast, the reconstruction was planned based on a contralateral augmentation to provide the best result. During the first stage a 400 cc expander was inserted. A second stage, left submuscular procedure was performed 6 months later. A 410 cc anatomic, textured implant with highly cohesive gel was inserted. The right breast was augmented with a 220 cc implant. Nipple reconstruction was performed 6 months after insertion of the final implants. Her postoperative results are good.

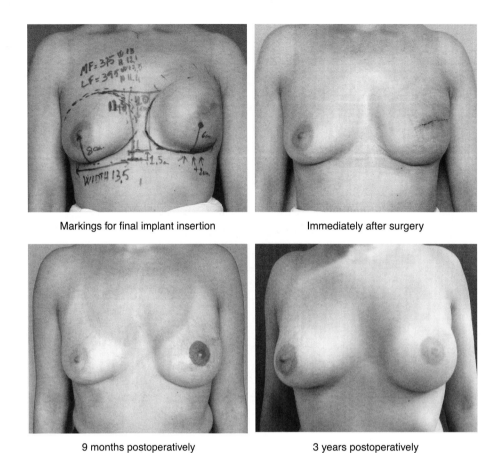

Markings for final implant insertion   Immediately after surgery

9 months postoperatively   3 years postoperatively

FIG. 13

This 34-year-old patient had a simple left mastectomy for DCIs. At the time of the mastectomy a two-stage immediate reconstruction was initiated. During the first stage a 400 cc expander was inserted. Six months later a 375 cc anatomic, textured implant with highly cohesive gel was inserted submuscularly. The size and the shape of the reconstructed left breast eliminated the need for surgery to the right breast. Six months after implant insertion she had nipple reconstruction, and 3 months following nipple reconstruction an areola tattoo was placed.

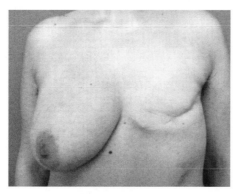

After mastectomy

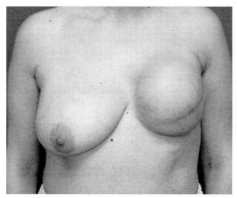

After expander insertion

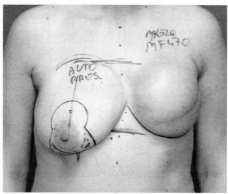

Final implant and contralateral reduction markings

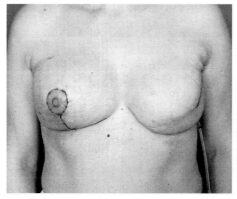

Immediately after surgery

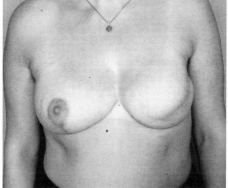

2 years postoperatively

FIG. 14

This 45-year-old patient had a simple left mastectomy for DCIs. A delayed two-stage reconstruction with contralateral reshaping was begun 4 years after the mastectomy. During the first stage a 500 cc expander was inserted. Six months later a 520 cc, anatomic, textured implant with highly cohesive gel was inserted submuscularly. The contralateral breast was reduced using an autoprosthesis technique whereby an inferior dermal-glandular pedicle was sutured to the pectoralis major to enhance the projection of the central area and to avoid a relapse of ptosis. A superior pedicle was used to supply the nipple-areola complex. The patient did not want nipple and areola reconstruction.

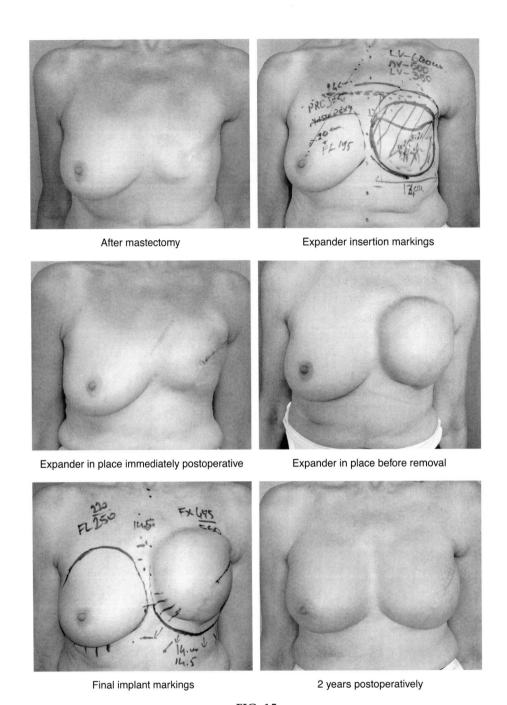

After mastectomy

Expander insertion markings

Expander in place immediately postoperative

Expander in place before removal

Final implant markings

2 years postoperatively

FIG. 15

This 62-year-old patient had a left simple mastectomy for DCIs with a two-stage, delayed reconstruction 6 years later. During the first stage a 500 cc, anatomic, medium-profile expander was inserted. Six months later the expander was removed, and a 615 cc, anatomic, textured implant with highly cohesive gel was placed submuscularly. A full-projection implant was used because the contralateral breast was augmented with a 235 cc implant. The patient did not want nipple and areola reconstruction and was satisfied with her postoperative result.

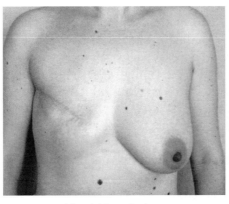
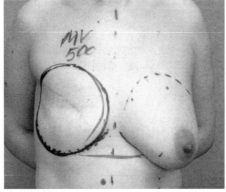

After right mastectomy   Expander insertion markings

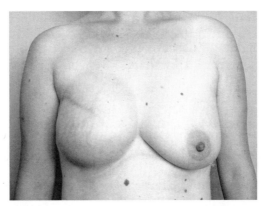

Before left mastectomy and removal of right expander

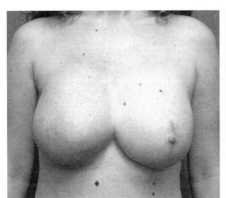
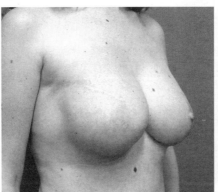
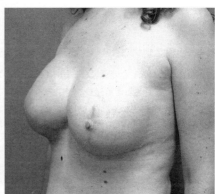

1 year postoperatively

FIG. 16

This 31-year-old patient had a right mastectomy for DCIs with a delayed two-stage re-construction after 2 years. At the time of the planned reconstruction, the patient showed a BRCA1-positive mutation. Therefore, a 500 cc anatomic expander was inserted, and a prophylactic left mastectomy with immediate one-stage reconstruction was planned for the time of the second stage procedure for the right breast. A 450 cc, submuscular, an-atomic, textured implant with highly cohesive gel was inserted on each side. Her post-operative result is acceptable.

CONCLUSION

Implants filled with highly cohesive silicone gel became commercially available in the 1990s, revolutionizing breast reconstruction. With the introduction of these new implants have come improved methods for determining proper implant volume; we have progressed from visual attempts to match the contralateral breast to a mathematic process. The contralateral breast is carefully measured to select a biodimensionally correct implant. It is essential for both immediate and delayed reconstruction to fully discuss expected results and possible complications with the patient. The surgeon must clearly envision the results to be achieved, including any possible contralateral procedure, to select the correct expander or permanent implant. The most important elements of a reconstructed breast are the inframammary fold, the inferior pole, the superior slope, and the projection. The inframammary fold and the inferior pole are related to accurate preoperative planning and appropriate surgical technique. Good superior slope and projection can be obtained using anatomic, textured implants filled with highly cohesive silicone gel. A prosthesis with a full projection can improve the outcome so that the results are more aesthetic. Anatomic implants filled with highly cohesive silicone gel are commercially available in many shapes to enable surgeons to individualize treatment for each patient.

SUGGESTED READINGS

Barone FE, Perry L, Keller T, et al. The biomechanical and histopathologic effects of surface texturing with silicone and polyurethane in tissue implantation and expansion. Plast Reconstr Surg 90:77, 1992.

Bayati S, Seckel BR. Inframammary crease ligament. Plast Reconstr Surg 95:501, 1995.

Beasley ME. Two stage expander/implant reconstruction: Delayed. In Spear SL, Little W, Lippman E, et al, eds. Surgery of the Breast: Principles and Art. Philadelphia: Lippincott, 1998.

Bostwick J III. Plastic and Reconstructive Breast Surgery. St Louis: Quality Medical Publishing, 1990.

Charpy A. Peauciers et aponévroses. In Traité d'Anatomie Humaine Publié sur la Direction de P. Poirier. Paris, 1896.

Chiarugi G. Istituzioni di Anatomia Dell'uomo. Milan, 1908.

Colen SR. Immediate two-stage breast reconstruction utilizing a tissue expander and implant. In Spear SL, Little W, Lippman E, et al, eds. Surgery of the Breast: Principles and Art. Philadelphia: Lippincott, 1998.

Cooper AP. On the Anatomy of the Breast. London: Longmans, 1940.

Dowden RV. Achieving a natural inframammary fold and ptotic effect in the reconstructed breast. Ann Plast Surg 19:524, 1987.

Francel TJ, Ryan JJ, Manson PN. Breast reconstruction utilizing implants: A local experience and comparison of three techniques. Plast Reconstr Surg 92:786, 1993.

Garnier D, Angonin R, Foulon P, et al. Le sillon sousmammaire: Mythe ou réalité? Ann Chir Plast Esthét 36:313, 1991.

Handel N, Jensen JA. An improved technique for creation of the inframammary fold in silicone implant breast reconstruction. Plast Reconstr Surg 89:558, 1992.

Lockwood TE. Superficial fascial system (SFS) of the trunk and extremities: A new concept. Plast Reconstr Surg 87:1009, 1991.

Maillard GF, Garey LJ. An improved technique for immediate retropectoral reconstruction after subcutaneous mastectomy. Plast Reconstr Surg 80:396, 1987.

Maillard GF, Montandon D, Goin J-L. Implant placed under an inversed abdominoplasty. In Maillard GF. Plastic Reconstructive Breast Surgery. Chicago: Year Book Medical, 1983, p 210.

Maxwell GP, Falcone PA. Eighty-four consecutive breast reconstructions using a textured silicone tissue expander. Plast Reconstr Surg 89:1022, 1992.

May JW Jr, Attwood J, Bartlett S. Staged use of soft-tissue expansion and lower thoracic advancement flap in breast reconstruction. Plast Reconstr Surg 79:272, 1987.

Nava M, Cortinovis U, Ottolenghi J, et al. Skin reducing mastectomy. Plast Reconstr Surg (submitted for publication).

Noone RB. Adjustable implant reconstruction. In Spear SL, Little W, Lippman E, et al, eds. Surgery of the Breast: Principles and Art. Philadelphia: Lippincott, 1998.

Pennisi VR. Making a definite inframammary fold under a reconstructed breast. Plast Reconstr Surg 60:523, 1977.

Pinella JW. Creating an inframammary crease with a liposuction cannula [letter]. Plast Reconstr Surg 83:925, 1989.

Querci della Rovere G, Benson JR, Breach N, et al, eds. Oncoplastic and Reconstructive Surgery of the Breast. London: Taylor & Francis, 2004.

Radovan C. Breast reconstruction after mastectomy using the temporary expander. Plast Reconstr Surg 69:195, 1982.

Rieffel H. L'appareil Génital de la Fémme. In Traité d'Anatomie Humaine Publié sur la Direction de P. Poirier et A. Paris, 1901.

Rosato RM, Dowden RV. Radiation therapy as a cause of capsular contracture. Ann Plast Surg 32:342, 1994.

Ryan JJ. A lower thoracic advancement flap in breast reconstruction after mastectomy. Plast Reconstr Surg 70:153, 1982.

Schuster RH, Kuske RR, Young VL, et al. Breast reconstruction in women treated with radiation therapy for breast cancer: Cosmesis, complications, and tumor control. Plast Reconstr Surg 90:445, 1992.

Sebileau P. Demonstrations d'Anatomie. Paris, 1892.

Slavin SA, Colen SR. Sixty consecutive breast reconstructions with the inflatable expander: A critical appraisal. Plast Reconstr Surg 86:910, 1990.

Spear SL. Primary implant reconstruction. In Spear SL, Little W, Lippman E, et al, eds. Surgery of the Breast: Principles and Art. Philadelphia: Lippincott, 1998.

Spear SL, Majidian A. Immediate breast reconstruction in two stages using textured, integrated-valve tissue expanders and breast implants: A retrospective review of 171 consecutive breast reconstructions from 1989 to 1996. Plast Reconstr Surg 101:53, 1998.

Spear SL, Spittler CJ. Breast reconstruction with implants and expanders. Plast Reconstr Surg 107:177, 2001.

Sterzi G. La Fascia superficiale. In Il Tessuto Sottocutaneo (Tela Subcutanea): Ricerhe Anatomiche. Florence, Italy, 1910, p 62.

van Straalen WH, Hage JJ, Bloemena E. The inframammary ligament: Myth or reality? Ann Plast Surg 35:237, 1995.

Versaci AD. A method of reconstructing a pendulous breast utilizing the tissue expander. Plast Reconstr Surg 80:387, 1987.

Editorial Commentary

This large European group has considerable experience using cohesive gel implants for immediate breast reconstruction. They start out by discussing the Becker expander permanent implant, which has been a very good appliance for breast reconstruction. It can be controlled in terms of size, and it can be very satisfactory for patients because they are involved in the decision-making. In fact, by using an external port, which in my own practice is frequently used, a patient can actually control the expansion or overexpansion of the appliance as indicated.

This article points out that reconstruction can be carried out relatively quickly using the cohesive implant, and when immediate reconstruction is not possible, the procedure can be carried out at a later date. The authors also point out that it is possible to perform delayed reconstruction by placing an expander first and placing the cohesive gel implant later. However, one point that is stressed, yet sometimes overlooked, is that there must be careful preoperative planning to ensure that the postoperative shape, size, and position are accurately assessed. If this is not carried out, then asymmetry can occur in all of these areas. When initial expansion of the breast is required, which is often the case in reconstructive techniques, then the necessary expansion should be maintained for 6 weeks before inserting the definitive implant. Once again it must be emphasized that the incision should be large enough for the implant to be placed without undue trauma, otherwise the procedure will undoubtedly result in an implant of an improper shape, which defeats the purpose of the cohesive gel implant.

Again it is stated that if one accepts a cohesive gel implant for use, there is probably a higher risk of capsule formation, and it may be necessary to do an open capsulotomy.

Although at the moment cohesive gel implants come in various sizes, they are obviously not comprehensive in terms of volume or shape. However, it is not inconceivable that in the near future there will be a method of manufacturing implants that can provide an exact match to contralateral breasts. Again, this will depend on popular demand. It is likely that this will be easier to accomplish with cohesive gel implants, because the technology certainly exists, and these implants naturally show greater stability in size and shape than previously used prostheses.

This article gives very good information and surgical steps for using either a one-stage or a two-stage reconstructive procedure. There will be more and more of an effort to produce the perfect breast form for unfortunate patients who have had to undergo a mastectomy.

Ian T. Jackson, MD

This excellent article summarizes the indications and techniques of one-stage and two-stage reconstruction using expansion. As in several of the other articles in this collection, the importance of measurement is raised as a method for achieving good results. Dr. Nava's team points out the importance of assessing the critical anatomic features that remain following mastectomy, and how to best use these to the advantage of the patient. The main elements of the preoperative assessment technique are reviewed, and step by step instructions are outlined. This group of authors has outlined the various devices that are marketed in a matrix of products. If most of these products did not exist, a busy surgeon would not miss them. Extremes of shape are problematic over the long run because of the adverse effects of biomechanical forces on tissues, and, in my opinion, they are best avoided. These authors correctly point out that although the goal of reconstruction was originally to create volume in the correct location to simplify the activities of daily living for cancer victims, the state of reconstruction has advanced to the point where we seek to achieve the goal of aesthetic reconstruction. In other words, our goal today is to provide mastectomy patients with breasts that look and feel as real as their natural breasts. This goal is of course not always achievable, but results today are several orders of magnitude better than they were 25 years ago. Further developments will allow even greater satisfaction as we get closer to providing an ideal result in every case.

Claudio De Lorenzi, BA, MD

Present Technology and Future Directions

Dennis C. Hammond, MD

The question of whether shaped breast implants offer any practical advantage in aesthetic and reconstructive breast surgery has proved difficult to answer. There are many reasons for this difficulty, and understanding these reasons is almost as important as understanding the devices themselves. Because breast implants come in various sizes, shapes, textures, and compositions, the many design variables involved make it difficult to draw reasonable conclusions about the performance of a given device. In addition, the approach an individual surgeon takes when using breast implants can have a profound effect on how each device ultimately performs. Just a few of the many variables involved here include patient selection, patient and surgeon expectations, preoperative appearance of the breast, and pocket location for the implant. Taken together, these issues allow almost any conclusion to be reached regarding which type of breast implant will perform best, with the most important variable often being the preconceived notions of the surgeon.

The previous articles in this monograph have documented the efficacy of shaped breast implants for providing outstanding results in both aesthetic and reconstructive breast surgery. The goal of this article is to briefly examine the history of anatomic implant designs, describe the progression of the anatomic shape concept, and discuss the future directions that implant designs might take.

ANATOMIC IMPLANT DESIGN

After the original smooth-walled silicone gel breast implant was developed in 1963 by Cronin and Gerow,[1] design modifications began to be introduced that aimed to improve the results provided by these devices. As a result, the first anatomically shaped implant appeared in the late 1960s as a smooth-walled silicone gel product that had a Dacron patch attached to the back of the device. Later versions of this device had five Dacron patches. The purpose of the patches was to initiate tissue ingrowth to help keep the device properly oriented. The shape of the device was aggressive—the upper pole had a relatively sharp angle, and most of the volume was located in the lower half (Fig. 1). The design of this device was conceptually brilliant. This was the first time the shape of an implant was designed to create a specific breast contour, rather than let the implant fold and wrinkle passively as dictated by the overlying breast. Even though this was new technology, the designers demonstrated surprisingly accurate imagination. Unfortunately, this device was associated with a very high rate of capsular contracture, and it

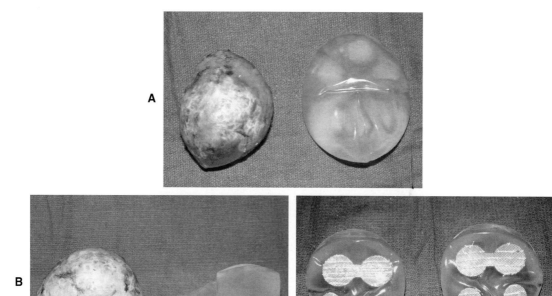

FIG. 1 **A** and **B,** Anteroposterior and lateral view of an early-design, shaped anatomic silicone gel implant before *(left)* and after *(right)* removal of a contracted capsule. **C,** With the implants turned over, the Dacron patches can be seen.

soon fell into disfavor. At the time it was felt that the Dacron patches somehow were responsible for the excessively high rate of capsular contracture. A saline alternative was eventually developed that had the same aggressive shape profile as the Dacron patched device; however, the shell was smooth, and there was no predictable way to ensure that the implant would not rotate and spoil the effect of the anatomic shape (Fig. 2).

The next significant step in anatomic implant design was the development of polyurethane-coated devices.[2] Two of these devices enjoyed significant popularity, the only difference between them being shape—the Meme implant (round) (Fig. 3, *A*) and the Replicon implant (shaped) (Fig. 3, *B*), both manufactured by Surgitek. The Replicon proved to be important in the history of breast implant development, because it was the first device manufactured with a textured surface. The polyurethane foam coating on these devices underwent a gradual biochemical degradation that created a low-grade inflammatory response in the capsule that formed around the device.[2] The result was a significant decrease in the rate of capsular contracture with these devices. In my own experience, the results obtained with these devices were some of the softest I have encountered. But what is more important, when using the Replicon device the interaction

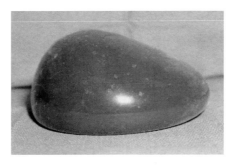

FIG. 2   An early-design, shaped saline implant. These devices were prone to malposition and rotation because the smooth surface provided no mechanism to hold them in the proper orientation.

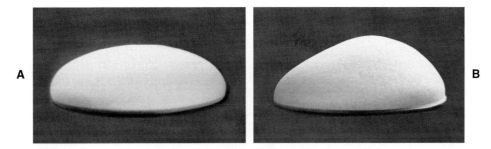

FIG. 3   **A,** Side view of the polyurethane foam–coated round Surgitek Meme silicone gel implant. **B,** Side view of the polyurethane foam–coated shaped Surgitek Replicon silicone gel implant.

between the capsule and the polyurethane foam coating prevented the implant from rotating. Thus the polyurethane foam coating served a dual purpose: preventing capsular contracture and fixing the implant in position.

One limitation of the Replicon device was that the shape was not as aggressive as earlier designs. As a result, a strategy employed at that time was to stack a smaller Meme implant on top of the lower pole of a larger Replicon device to increase overall projection and create a more shaped construct.[2] This was a very forward-thinking concept and was made possible by the textured polyurethane surface that tended to hold the two devices in position. Unfortunately, uncertainties arose about the polyurethane surface and the breakdown products of the foam-lattice network, and claims were made that these breakdown products were carcinogenic. Subsequent scientific work disputed these claims, but the manufacturer of these devices withdrew from the implant market. Recently several European and South American companies have had some success reintroducing devices coated with polyurethane foam. Whether these devices can ultimately regain access to the U.S. market remains to be seen. However, the benefits demonstrated by the shape concepts used in these early devices were largely responsible for the advances that followed.

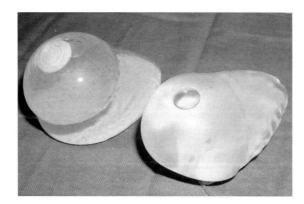

FIG. 4   Oblique view of a stacked tissue expander *(left)*, which was essentially two expanders with separate valves. The expander on top was designed to preferentially expand the lower pole of the breast. The differential expander *(right)* was designed to accomplish the same task because the thinner and more pliant silicone envelope in the lower half of the device allowed the lower pole to balloon out as it expanded.

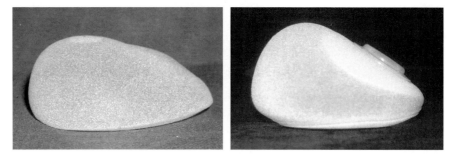

FIG. 5   Lateral view of two different versions of anatomically shaped textured tissue expanders with integrated valves for inflation.

The next significant advance in shaped design came with the development of shaped tissue expanders. This development was fueled by the concept that, after mastectomy, the skin envelope could be differentially expanded to prepare for placement of an implant. To this end, devices designed by Manders, Fisher, and Maxwell in the late 1980s all provided evidence that the shape of an expander could effectively influence the shape of the breast during expansion (Figs. 4 and 5). The shapes of tissue expanders used most commonly today are still influenced by the early designs (Fig. 6).

Another design feature introduced with these expanders was silicone texturing on the surface. Several types of textured surfaces were developed, all attempting to reduce the rate of capsular contracture as noted with polyurethane foam.[3] The effect of surface texturing on the breast capsule proved to be mainly structural, because a capsule integrates itself into the surface of an implant as dictated by the aggressiveness of the texture. However, the inflammatory response noted with polyurethane has not been seen with silicone texturing. Therefore the results of clinical studies have been mixed regarding the

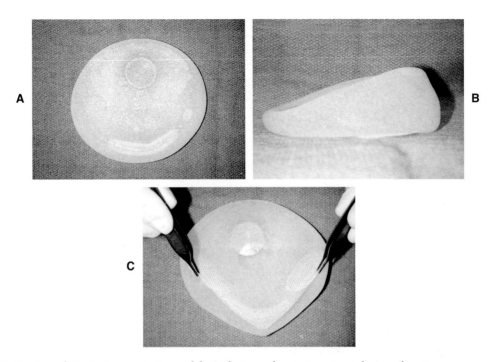

FIG. 6　**A** and **B**, Anteroposterior and lateral view of a more recent design showing an aggressive shape with a textured surface. **C**, Two reinforced tabs at the base of the device allow the expander to be sutured in position to prevent postoperative rotation.

effect of silicone surface texturing in relation to the development of capsular contracture. Whether these textured surfaces actually decrease the rate of capsular contracture can be argued, but one unique feature of the most aggressive textures is tissue ingrowth. As collagen fibers form around the implant, the open pore network of the textured surface creates a three-dimensional structure that is variably penetrated by the capsule, creating a semirigid, Velcrolike bond. This "bond" between the capsule and the textured surface occurs more consistently and more completely with tissue expanders than with implants because the pressure in the tissue expander pushes the textured surface into the capsule, helping to ensure maximal contact and enhancing the chances for capsule ingrowth into the interstices of the textured surface. Although the effect of tissue ingrowth on reducing the rate of capsular contracture remains uncertain, one very beneficial result of this interaction between the implant surface and the capsule is that the implant is locked into position when ingrowth occurs. Even if no ingrowth develops, a textured surface still provides an element of friction that helps the implant resist rotation.

Further advancement in breast implant design slowed significantly because of controversy related to the safety of silicone gel. Although subsequent scientific work documented benign interaction of silicone with the body, the use of implants filled with silicone gel was restricted to only a few investigators. Practically speaking, the only devices available for use in breast surgery in the United States through all of the 1990s were filled with saline. Despite this limitation, the utility of shaped implants continued to be investigated as it applied to saline implants. Several different implants were developed,

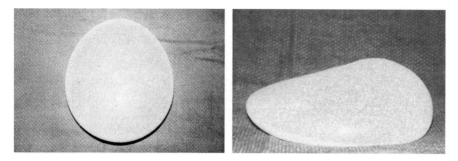

FIG. 7   Anteroposterior and lateral view of a shaped saline implant, tall height design.

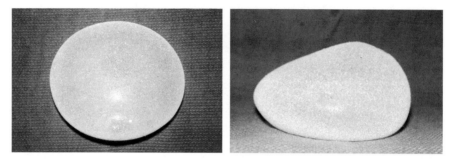

FIG. 8   Anteroposterior and lateral view of a shaped saline implant, short height design.

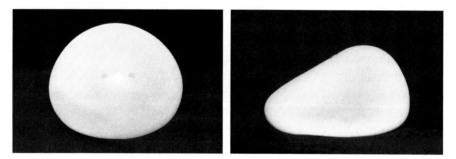

FIG. 9   Anteroposterior and lateral view of a more aggressively shaped saline implant, short height design.

and an attempt was made to correlate shape and implant height. Ultimately several different devices were developed with differing heights and projections (Figs. 7 through 9). The major drawback of these devices relates to the characteristics of the saline fill. To avoid the shell wrinkling associated with underfilling any saline implant, particularly when placed upright, considerable attention to the degree of implant fill is required, and there is a real tendency to slightly overfill these devices to avoid this problem. This filling tendency is a detriment to the device's shape, because the aggressiveness of the shape diminishes with increased volume. Specifically, the upper pole of a shaped saline im-

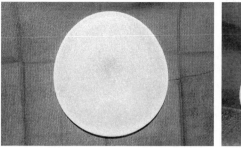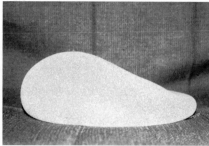

FIG. 10   Anteroposterior and lateral view of a minimally cohesive anatomically shaped silicone gel implant with an aggressive shape.

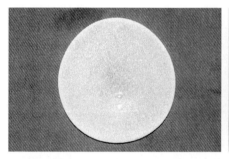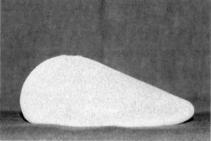

FIG. 11   Anteroposterior and lateral view of a strongly cohesive anatomically shaped silicone gel implant with an aggressive shape.

plant tends to develop an increasingly convex contour as the volume increases so that, if one is overfilled too much, it differs little from a round implant. For this reason, many surgeons have questioned not only the utility of these devices, but also the validity of using anatomic shapes.

As restrictions have eased on silicone gel devices, lessons learned over the past 30 years have been applied to a new generation of devices. These shaped silicone gel implants fall generally into two categories based on the cohesiveness of the gel used to fill them. Several relatively noncohesive, aggressively shaped, textured silicone gel implants were introduced for use in aesthetic and reconstructive breast surgery (Fig. 10). Later a much more cohesive line of textured gel-filled devices was introduced, again with an aggressive shape (Fig. 11). The more-cohesive devices were designed to offer several different heights and projections. The previous articles in this monograph have documented the results obtained using these devices. Of all the shaped devices developed over the past 30 years, these shaped silicone gel implants have provided, in my experience, the best and most consistent aesthetic results I have seen in both aesthetic and reconstructive breast surgery. Specifically, they offer precise control of the upper pole of the breast.

The less-cohesive shaped gel implants are softer than the more-cohesive gel implants and, given that they are less crosslinked, tend to wrinkle, because the gel cannot fully support the outer shell of the device, particularly when the implant is placed upright. This wrinkling can be visible in patients with a thin, soft tissue envelope. Studies of

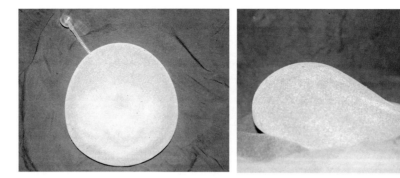

FIG. 12   Anteroposterior and lateral view of an anatomically shaped implant with a combination of a gel outer lumen and a saline inner lumen. The fill valve and tubing can be seen.

these devices are ongoing to determine what considerations may become important in the future. However, the cohesive devices, because of the more stable support of the implant shell, resist wrinkling and allow much more aggressive shapes to be created. With these devices the implant provides most of the breast shape. When a device is properly chosen with respect to length, width, and projection, the results can be outstanding. The gel used in these implants is so cohesive that rupture is eliminated as a complication—the significance of this advantage cannot be overstated. However, it must be noted that these newer, more cohesive, shaped devices are associated with some of their own problems. Issues such as implant rotation despite using textured surfaces must be addressed. Interestingly, cases of gel fracture have also been noted wherein cohesive devices have been inserted through incisions that are too small. In these instances the outer shell of the implant remains intact, but the shape of the device is altered because of a disruption in the internal cohesive gel. When gel fracture is noted during insertion, it is advisable to replace the altered implant and enlarge the incision to allow a new device to be inserted without injuring it.

THE FUTURE

Although significant improvements in implant design have clearly been made, further design modifications are on the horizon. Improvements in shape, size, and projection will undoubtedly be forthcoming as experience grows with these devices. Manipulating the cohesive nature of the gel will likely provide softer devices and yet allow sufficient support to prevent wrinkling. Also, issues regarding patient selection and how to use these implants optimally will become better defined.

One new concept that has emerged in European studies involves a combination gel and saline device that incorporates texture and an anatomic shape with the ability to moderately adjust its volume. This device uses relatively cohesive gel and has an inner saline bladder fixed to the lower pole (Fig. 12). A remote fill tube is used to add saline as needed. Early results are encouraging, although it remains uncertain when such a device may become generally available in the United States.

CONCLUSION

Surgeons and manufacturers have been developing modifications to shape, texture, dimension, and fill of implants, manipulating each variable to produce the highest quality devices that achieve the best possible results for aesthetic and reconstructive breast surgery. As we emerge from the cloud created by the controversy of silicone gel safety, the quality of these devices will only improve—and the future is indeed bright.

REFERENCES

1. Cronin TD, Gerow FJ. Augmentation mammaplasty: A new "natural feel" prosthesis. Exerpta Medica International Congress Series 66:41, 1963.
2. Hester TR Jr, Nahai F, Bostwick J, et al. A 5-year experience with polyurethane-covered mammary prostheses for treatment of capsular contracture, primary augmentation mammoplasty, and breast reconstruction. Clin Plast Surg 15:569-585, 1988.
3. Maxwell GP, Hammond DC. Breast implants: Smooth versus textured. In Habal MB, Woods JE, Morain WD, et al, eds. Advances in Plastic and Reconstructive Surgery, vol 9. St Louis: Mosby, 1993, pp 209-220.

Editorial Commentary

This article is a useful reminder of what breast implant technology is available at the moment and what can be expected in the future when we look back on the road we have traveled and the implant modifications that have been introduced. We see that this road has sometimes been a rocky one. Changes in implant design have been frequent and often instituted for the wrong reasons—especially when resulting from ill-considered government intervention. Fortunately, as a result of the vast experience of surgeons outside of the United States, we can publish results on cohesive implants. In addition to this, we in the United States will be able to use these implants safely because of the experience of our European colleagues. This has placed us in a favorable position that is well-documented in Dr. Hammond's contribution.

Not only have surgeons benefited from these developments but our patients have as well. When cohesive gel implants become freely available we will be able to offer our patients a safe, satisfactory product that is unlikely to cause local problems and is long lasting. However, as pointed out in this article, this is not the end of the line—it is probably the beginning of a new line. Research and development will continue until eventually the truly ideal implant will emerge.

Ian T. Jackson, MD

Dr. Hammond outlines the history of breast implant devices to the present day and then looks beyond to outline possibilities for the future. This excellent summary gives the reader a sense of why things are as they are today. Dr. Hammond provides the reader with valuable background information that creates perspective for surgeons. In his opening paragraph, Dr. Hammond indicates his uncertainty regarding whether shaped cohesive III devices offer any practical advantage. This may be because U.S. surgeons have been severely restricted in their device choices since 1992. Surgeons who have workaday experience with third generation cohesive gel devices routinely tout their advantages in various situations.

Dr. Hammond also reviews the history of texture applied to devices, noting that currently available textures were developed by trying to emulate the success of polyurethane foam in attenuating the scourge of capsular contracture. Various texture-creating processes have been tried, but two main types have survived. One takes an imprint of polyurethane foam by pressing a sheet of silicone against a sheet of foam, whereas the other uses a salt-loss technique to create a more aggressive, higher-friction surface.* Neither surface typically allows tissue ingrowth (so-called *Velcro adhesion*) during routine implant use. An exception to this occurs with Biocell devices (with salt-loss texture) under high pressures, as in tissue expansion. In my experience, this phenomenon is not typically seen with either surface in routine uncomplicated breast implant use.†

In addition, Dr. Hammond raises the very important issue of device malrotation. Shaped devices risk a type of complication that simply does not exist in round devices.‡ A shaped device that rotates in the pocket results in an odd shape, because the upper pole projection is too great. I have seen this unfortunate complication with both Siltex and Biocell implants. Trying to find reasons for malrotation in some cases and not others creates consternation and frustration. However, in my experience, common causes for malrotation (after the implant has been properly inserted) are inadequate or improper pocket dissection (surgeon factors); undue external pressure, such as patients sleeping with their arms under their breasts (patient factors); and the coefficient of friction of the surface of the device (device factors). Any of these causes may result in malrotation,§ and the surgeon should keep these in mind when counseling patients and using these implants.

*There are primarily two different approaches to manufacturing implant texture. The first involves pressing processed silicone sheets against a sheet of foam under pressure creating a "foam print," much like creating a footprint while walking. The original process was acquired by Mentor and forms the basis for the Siltex surface. On the other hand, the salt loss technique involves a different strategy. Silicone shells are dipped in liquid silicone dispersion and are then sprinkled with salt crystals, partially cured, redipped, and finally rubbed so that the salt crystals are partially exposed. After washing, the salt crystals dissolve, leaving behind their angular shapes permanently cast in the silicone shell. This more aggressive texturing is used by Inamed in their Biocell surface.

†A curious phenomenon is sometimes seen when a layer of tissue coats the Biocell surface, which itself becomes the new interface with the implant pocket. In my experience, this capsule within a capsule phenomenon is typically only seen with the Biocell surface, not the Siltex, but this type of inner capsule is not unusual in Biocell devices. There sometimes is some adherence at the upper pole, and the inner capsule is less well formed at the inferior pole.

‡Infrequently, round devices may flip back to front, and, depending on the degree of silicone crosslinking present, may be visible in some patients. This problem is not easily seen with low crosslinked devices, because they tend to assume the shape of the pocket they reside in and respond to gravity by flowing to the lowest points.

§Creating an adequate, precisely shaped pocket helps prevent rotational pressures that would cause a device to rotate. Shaped devices are heavier at the bottom, so that patients with malrotation sometimes have spontaneous correction after being upright.

Dr. Hammond also correctly points out that wrinkling of an implant is an important issue and that, as surgeons, we want to avoid evident wrinkling on the surface of the breast at rest. Whether an implant wrinkles depends on several factors, implant factors being only one subset of the universe of causes. I have seen wrinkling with all devices, regardless of manufacturing technique, and in all implant locations—even in patients that were appropriately selected.* Wrinkling of devices is related to the quality, quantity, and location of the skin, fat, and parenchyma, and the pressure applied to the surface of the implant by the tissues. An implant on the table is subject to atmospheric pressure, but an implant in situ is subject to other pressures (natural breast weight, muscle activity, and so on). Additionally, remember that the breast is dynamic: it moves, and the manner in which these devices respond to acceleration forces is also an important factor of wrinkling. Also keep in mind that devices with less crosslinking may be prone to more wrinkling, as are patients with thinner skin, less parenchyma, and less fat.

These authors have written a very concise review of a very complex issue. Hopefully the reader is stimulated to read more on this fascinating topic and perhaps contribute to our knowledge base to help give our patients even better results.

Claudio De Lorenzi, BA, MD

---

*If the definition of *wrinkling* is "regular undulations visible on the surface of the breast," then I have also seen wrinkling in breasts without implants (such as when patients are asked to bend over and let their breasts hang downwards—the weight of the parenchyma pulls the skin and sometimes causes tension wrinkling of the upper pole).

Continuing Medical Education

Continuing Medical Education
Post Test Questions

Please complete this Post Test by circling the correct answer on the Answer Sheet that follows. You must achieve a score of 70% or greater in order to have demonstrated understanding of the content.

1. Which of the following best describe the factors determining success in breast augmentation with cohesive gel breast implants?
   a. The thickness of the chest skin that will cover the proposed implant
   b. The thickness of the subcutaneous fatty layer
   c. The thickness of the patient's natural breast parenchyma
   d. All of the above

2. Physical examination of a patient undergoing evaluation for breast augmentation may be entirely conducted with the patient supine and one breast uncovered at a time.
   a. True
   b. False

3. Which of the following best describes the expected increase in bra cup size per 200 cc of breast implant volume?
   a. 1 cup
   b. 2 cups
   c. 3 cups
   d. It depends on the size of the patient

4. Periareolar incisions are not appropriate if the areolar diameter is less than 35 mm.
   a. True
   b. False

5. Patients with more pigment in their skin are better candidates for periareolar augmentation.
   a. True
   b. False

6. (Choose all that are correct.) The sternalis muscle:
   a. Is found above the pectoralis major muscle
   b. Is found beneath the pectoralis major muscle
   c. Has vertical fibers extending from the manubrium to the 6th or 7th costal cartilages
   d. Is found in approximately 4% of the population
   e. Is found in approximately 40% of the population

7. In breast reconstruction using anatomic cohesive-gel implants and the omental flap, which statement is incorrect?
   a. The omental flap is easy to shape
   b. The omental flap's blood supply is abundant and safe
   c. The omental flap reaches the mastectomy site without tension because of the length of its pedicle
   d. The consistency of the omental flap is not similar to breast tissue
   e. The omental flap may be harvested laparoscopically and without a complementary epigastric incision

8. In some patients, harvesting part of the pectoralis major muscle (segmental pectoralis major muscle flap) may be necessary to help conceal the implant's borders in the superior/medial pole of the breast. Which of the statements below is incorrect?
   a. This technique is generally used for very thin patients or for those requesting larger implants
   b. The segmental pectoralis major muscle flap is placed along and over the implant's superomedial pole without any fixation
   c. The segmental pectoralis major muscle flap is based on perforators located along the sternal border
   d. Lateral/superior dislocation of an implant resulting from contraction of the pectoralis muscle is avoided because only a strip of the muscle is used
   e. The flap is generally 15 cm long and 4 cm wide

9. In primary breast augmentation using cohesive-gel implants, which of the following is true?
   a. The pectoralis fascia is attached to the sternum and the clavicle, and it is not continuous with the fascia of the shoulder, axilla, and thorax inferolaterally
   b. When using the inframammary approach, the incision is usually 4 cm long and should always be located slightly medial to the inferior projection of the nipple-areola complex on the inframammary fold
   c. When using the periareolar approach, the incision should always be placed along the inferior border of the areola
   d. Anatomic, cohesive, silicone-gel implants have a less natural shape, and their use decreases the chances of capsular contracture, rupture, and rippling
   e. With the subfascial approach, the stronger supporting system offered by the thickened fascia in the superior and medial regions of the breast improves the coverage and concealment of the implant borders in these areas

10. Which of the following types of implants were at one time stacked in an attempt to create more breast projection?
    a. Textured saline implants
    b. Polyurethane foam coated implants
    c. Anatomic gel implants
    d. None of the above

11. Each of the following is true of cohesive gel implants except:
    a. They have a tendency to form visible wrinkles
    b. They may be formed into aggressive shapes
    c. They are available only in conjunction with textured surfaces
    d. They provide excellent shape control of the upper pole of the breast

12. Anatomic saline implants:
    a. Must be underfilled to function properly
    b. Are available in only one height
    c. Tend to become convex in the upper pole as the implant becomes overfilled
    d. Can be sutured into position

13. Each of the following influenced the development of shaped implants except:
    a. Polyurethane foam–coated devices
    b. Shaped tissue expanders
    c. Cohesive silicone gel
    d. All of the above

14. Which fill material provides the firmest breast?
    a. Cohesive gel I
    b. Cohesive gel II
    c. Cohesive gel III
    d. Saline

15. What two components are important for the integrity of the implant shell?
    a. Surface pattern
    b. Gel consistency
    c. Material strength
    d. Optimal thickness

16. Rupture of a cohesive gel implant is best diagnosed by?
    a. Palpation
    b. Change in breast shape
    c. MRI scan
    d. Change in breast size

17. Which implants cause less capsule formation?
    a. Saline-filled implants
    b. Smooth gel-filled implants
    c. Cohesive gel implants
    d. Becker implants

18. What is the major disadvantage of less-cohesive gels?
   a. The breast becomes too firm
   b. Breast shape is not well maintained
   c. Development of wrinkles
   d. Early rupture of the implant

19. Which parameter(s) of textured implants filled with highly cohesive silicone gel is (are) the most important?
   a. Height
   b. Diameter
   c. Projection
   d. Volume

20. Is a mammography reliable in a reconstructed breast containing a textured implant filled with highly cohesive silicone gel?
   a. Always
   b. Never
   c. If the implant is beneath the muscle
   d. If the implant is above the muscle

21. The complication rate of reconstruction using an implant after radiotherapy is:
   a. <5%
   b. 10% to 20%
   c. 20% to 30%
   d. >50%

22. Using the serratus fascia to cover the lateral part of the textured implant filled with highly cohesive silicone gel is an important step of:
   a. The second stage of delayed reconstruction
   b. The second stage of immediate reconstruction
   c. One-stage immediate breast reconstruction

23. Silicone implants are contraindicated by which of the following?
   a. Patient has a silicone allergy
   b. Patient is less than 18 years of age
   c. Patient has a family history of breast cancer
   d. Patient has a very small breast
   e. Patient engages in a high level of exercise

24. What determines the size of an implant?
   a. The size of the areola
   b. The projection of the breast
   c. The width of the breast
   d. The grade of ptosis
   e. The patient

25. Which of the following instruments is not useful during an inframammary augmentation?
    a. Long scissor
    b. Long cautery
    c. Lighted hook
    d. Dissector
    e. Head light

26. Which of the following is not included in the "no touch" technique?
    a. Change of gloves
    b. Checking of the envelope integrity by the nurse
    c. Plastic bag for implant insertion
    d. Iodine solution
    e. Disinfection of the skin incision

27. Which of the following would necessitate an implant change?
    a. Hematoma
    b. Seroma
    c. Wound infection
    d. 10-year-old implant
    e. Wrong size implant

Innovations

IN PLASTIC SURGERY

Cohesive Gel Implants

Volume 1 • Number 3 • 2007

United States and international readers: To receive CME credit, please mail or fax payment of $25 along with completed Registration, Post Test, and Evaluation forms to: *Ciné-Med, Inc., CME Department, 127 Main Street North, Woodbury, CT 06798. Fax: 203-263-4839.*

REGISTRATION

Name _____

Address _____

Address _____

City _____ State / Zip _____

Phone _____ Fax _____

E-mail _____

Specialty _____

PAYMENT INFORMATION

CME Credit Fee: $25

____Check enclosed *(payable to Ciné-Med, Inc.)* ____VISA ____MasterCard ____American Express

Credit Card No. _____ Exp. Date _____

Authorized Signature _____

CME POST TEST ANSWER SHEET

1. a b c d
2. a b
3. a b c d
4. a b
5. a b
6. a b c d e
7. a b c d e

8. a b c d e
9. a b c d e
10. a b c d
11. a b c d
12. a b c d
13. a b c d
14. a b c d

15. a b c d
16. a b c d
17. a b c d
18. a b c d
19. a b c d
20. a b c d
21. a b c d

22. a b c
23. a b c d e
24. a b c d e
25. a b c d e
26. a b c d e
27. a b c d e

Innovations

IN PLASTIC SURGERY

Cohesive Gel Implants

Volume 1 • Number 3 • 2007

EVALUATION

Please rate each question on a scale of 5 to 1, with 5 being the highest and 1 being the lowest.

1. Objectives: To what extent were the objectives achieved?

	Excellent				Poor
a. Describe how to use cohesive gel implants for different body types.	5	4	3	2	1
b. Explain the step-by-step techniques for various breast reconstruction procedures.	5	4	3	2	1
c. Discuss the current status of cohesive gel implants in the marketplace.	5	4	3	2	1
d. Identify ways to embrace new devices and products while ensuring the safety of patients.	5	4	3	2	1

2. Content: To what extent did the program:

	Excellent				Poor
a. Increase your knowledge of the topic?	5	4	3	2	1
b. Present clear and organized content?	5	4	3	2	1
c. Meet your personal/educational objectives?	5	4	3	2	1
d. Help to improve patient care?	5	4	3	2	1
e. Cause you to make changes in your practice?	5	4	3	2	1

If you felt the content was *not* free of commercial bias, please explain:_____

_____

_____

3. Overall activity: 5   4   3   2   1

4. How long did it take you to complete this program? _____

Are there any educational topics that are not being sufficiently addressed? _____

_____

_____

_____

United States and international readers: To receive CME credit, please mail or fax payment of $25 along with completed Registration, Post Test, and Evaluation forms to: *Ciné-Med, Inc.,* *CME Department, 127 Main Street North, Woodbury, CT 06798. Fax: 203-263-4839.*

Notes

Notes

Notes

Notes